Caring for Life

St. John Ambulance Association

British Red Cross

Pocket
First Aid

St. John Ambulance
Dr Tony Lee KStJ MA BM BCh DObstRCOG Chief Medical Officer
Dr Lotte Newman CBE FRCGP FRNZCGP BSc Medical Adviser

St. Andrew's Ambulance Association
Mr Rudy Crawford BSc (Hons) MB ChB FRCS (Glasg) FFAEM
Chairman of Medical and First Aid Committee

British Red Cross
Dr J Gordon Paterson FFPHM FRCPE DRCOG DCM Chief Medical Adviser
Dr Vivien J Armstrong FRCA DRCOG PGCE Project Manager

DK

LONDON, NEW YORK, MUNICH,
MELBOURNE, DELHI

SENIOR EDITOR Janet Mohun
ART EDITOR Sara Freeman
DTP DESIGNER Julian Dams
SENIOR MANAGING EDITOR Jemima Dunne
MANAGING ART EDITOR Louise Dick
PRODUCTION CONTROLLER Louise Daly
PRODUCTION MANAGER Sarah Coltman

Produced for Dorling Kindersley by
COOLING BROWN
9–11 High St, Hampton, Middlesex TW12 2SA

Second edition first published in Great Britain in 2003
by Dorling Kindersley Limited, 80 Strand,
London WC2R 0RL
A Penguin Company

2 4 6 8 10 9 7 5 3 1

Illustration copyright © 2003 by
Dorling Kindersley Limited

Text copyright © 2003 by St. John Ambulance;
St. Andrew's Ambulance Association; The British
Red Cross Society

All enquiries regarding any extracts or re-use of
any material in this book should be addressed to the
publishers, Dorling Kindersley Limited

A CIP catalogue record for this book is available
from the British Library

ISBN 0 7513 4732 9 (Paperback)

Reproduced in Singapore by Colourscan
Printed and bound by South China
Printing Co. Ltd., China

For further information about the First Aid
Manual and Pocket First Aid visit:
www.dk.com/firstaidmanual

See our complete catalogue at
www.dk.com

CONTENTS

INTRODUCTION 4

1 TECHNIQUES AND EQUIPMENT 7

Monitoring vital signs 8
First-aid materials......................................10
Cold compresses 12
Sterile dressings..13
Principles of bandaging...............................14
Triangular bandages 16
Reef knots..16
Arm sling...17
Elevation sling..18

2 LIFE-SAVING PROCEDURES 19

Life-saving priorities 20
Adult resuscitation techniques 21
Child resuscitation techniques................32
Infant resuscitation techniques................40
Choking 45
Choking adult...46
Choking child...47
Choking infant..48

3 CIRCULATORY AND RESPIRATORY PROBLEMS 49

Shock 50
Anaphylactic shock 52
Angina pectoris...53
Acute heart failure.....................................53
Heart attack 54
Fainting...55
Asthma..56
Drowning...57
Penetrating chest wound.........................58

4 WOUNDS AND BLEEDING 59

Severe bleeding 60
Cuts and grazes...62
Foreign object in a cut.................................63

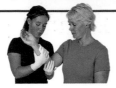

Scalp and head wounds......................64
Eye wound..65
Bleeding from the ear........................65
Nosebleed..66
Abdominal wound..............................67
Wound to the palm............................68
Wound at a joint crease......................68

5 BONE, JOINT, AND MUSCLE INJURIES 69

Types of injury..................................70
Strains and sprains............................72
Cheekbone and nose fractures............73
Fractured collar bone........................74
Shoulder injury................................75
Arm injury..76
Elbow injury....................................77
Hand and finger injuries....................78
Spinal injury....................................79
Fractured pelvis................................82
Hip and thigh injuries........................83
Knee injury......................................84
Lower leg injury................................85
Ankle injury......................................86
Foot and toe injuries........................86

6 DISORDERS OF CONSCIOUSNESS 87

Concussion......................................88
Cerebral compression........................89
Skull fracture..................................90
Stroke..91
Diabetes mellitus..............................92
Hyperglycaemia................................92
Hypoglycaemia................................93
Seizures in adults..............................94
Absence seizures..............................95
Seizures in children..........................96

7 ENVIRONMENTAL INJURIES 97

Severe burns and scalds....................98
Minor burns and scalds....................100
Burns to the airway..........................101
Electrical burn................................102
Chemical burn................................103
Chemical burn to the eye..................104
Heat exhaustion..............................105
Heatstroke....................................106
Frostbite..107
Hypothermia..................................108

8 FOREIGN OBJECTS 111

Splinter..112
Embedded fish-hook........................113
Foreign object in the eye..................114
Foreign object in the ear..................115
Foreign object in the nose................115
Inhaled foreign object......................116
Swallowed foreign object..................116

9 POISONING, BITES, AND STINGS 117

Swallowed poisons..........................118
Drug poisoning................................119
Alcohol poisoning............................120
Food poisoning................................121
Insect sting....................................122
Tick bite..122
Snake bite......................................123
Animal bite....................................124

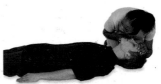

Index and acknowledgments..............125
Observation chart............................128

INTRODUCTION

This second edition of *Pocket First Aid* covers essential first-aid techniques in detail but in a compact format that is more readily accessible at a medical emergency. The book gives clear and comprehensive step-by-step advice on first-aid treatments, from life-saving resuscitation procedures to the dressing of wounds.

The information in this book has been taken from the revised 8th edition of the *First Aid Manual* written by the same authors and published by Dorling Kindersley. Advice has been based on guidelines agreed and issued internationally in

2001 for first-aid treatments and resuscitation techniques. The material in this manual provides guidance on initial care and treatment but should not be regarded as a substitute for medical advice.

The Voluntary Aid Societies do not accept responsibility for any claims arising from the use of this manual when the guidelines given have not been followed.

First aiders are advised to make sure that they keep up to date with developments, recognise the limits of their competence, and to obtain first-aid training from a qualified trainer.

HOW TO USE THIS BOOK

Colour bars help you to find relevant sections quickly

Introductory text describes likely causes and effects of condition

"Your aims" box summarises purposes of treatment

Annotated photographs show details of particular techniques

Steps explain each stage of first aid action

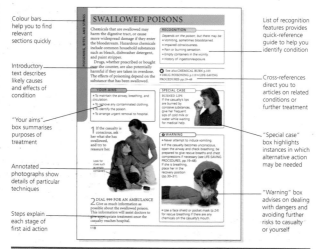

List of recognition features provides quick-reference guide to help you identify condition

Cross-references direct you to articles on related conditions or further treatment

"Special case" box highlights instances in which alternative action may be needed

"Warning" box advises on dealing with dangers and avoiding further risks to casualty or yourself

ACTION AT AN EMERGENCY

By working to a clear plan, you will be able to prioritise the demands that may be made on you in any emergency situation. Avoid placing yourself in danger, be aware of hazards such as petrol or gas, and do not attempt to do too much by yourself.

FIRST-AID PRIORITIES

● *Assess the situation.* Quickly and calmly observe what has happened, and look for dangers to yourself, to the casualty, and to bystanders. Consider whether anyone's life is in immediate danger; if there are bystanders who could help; and whether you need specialist help.

● *Make the area safe.* Conditions that gave rise to the incident may present a danger. Put your own safety first. Simple measures, such as turning off a switch, can often make the area safe.

● *Give emergency aid.* Assess all casualties to determine treatment priorities, and treat those with life-threatening conditions first. Establish whether the casualty is conscious, check whether his airway is open and whether he is breathing, and look for signs of circulation.

● *Get help from others.* Check that any necessary medical aid or other expert help has been called and is on its way.

TELEPHONING FOR HELP

You can summon help by telephone from a number of sources.

● **Emergency services** (dial 999): police, fire, and ambulance services; mine, mountain, cave, and fell rescue; HM Coastguard. Alternatively, you can ring 112, which is the European Union emergency number.

● **Utilities**: gas, electricity, or water.

● **Health services**: doctor, dentist, nurse, midwife, or NHS Direct (NHS phone and internet information service).

Emergency calls are free and can be made on any telephone, including car phones and mobile phones.

WHAT TO TELL EMERGENCY SERVICES

State your name, that you are a first aider, and give the following details:

● Your telephone number.

● The location of the incident; give a road name or number, if possible.

● The type of incident; for example, "Traffic accident, two cars, road blocked, three people trapped".

● The number, sex, and approximate ages of the casualties, and what you know about their condition.

● Details of any hazards or weather conditions, such as fog or ice.

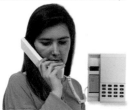

Phoning the emergency services
Try to stay calm so that you can give all the information the emergency services need. Do not hang up until the control officer has cleared the line.

LOOKING AFTER YOURSELF

When giving first aid, particularly if you are treating open wounds, it is important to prevent "cross infection" (transmitting germs to a casualty or contracting an infection yourself).

Often, simple measures, such as washing your hands and wearing disposable gloves, will provide sufficient protection. There is a risk of infection with blood-borne viruses such as hepatitis B or C and Human Immunodeficiency Virus (HIV), but these viruses can only be transmitted by blood-to-blood contact – if an infected person's blood makes contact with yours through, for example, a cut or graze.

Protection from hepatitis B
All first aiders should be protected against hepatitis B by immunisation. The vaccine is given as a series of three injections in the upper arm.

IMMUNISATION
It is recommended that all first aiders are immunised against hepatitis B. Currently, there is no vaccine against hepatitis C or HIV. If you think you have been exposed to any infection after giving first aid, seek medical aid immediately.

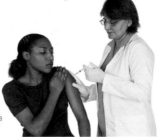

GUIDELINES FOR PREVENTING CROSS INFECTION

Following good practice guidelines will help to prevent infection.
• If possible, wash your hands in soap and water before treating a casualty.
• Carry protective disposable gloves with you and use them when you are giving treatment. If gloves are not available, ask the casualty to dress his own wound, or enclose your hands in clean plastic bags.
• Cover cuts and grazes on your hands with waterproof dressings.
• Wear a plastic apron when dealing with quantities of body fluids and plastic glasses to protect your eyes.
• Avoid touching a wound or any part of a dressing that will come into contact with a wound.

• Try not to breathe, cough, or sneeze over a wound while treating a casualty.
• Be extremely careful not to prick yourself with any needle found on or near a casualty or cut yourself on glass.
• If a face shield or pocket mask is available, use it when you are giving rescue breaths (p.24).
• Dispose of waste safely. Place soiled items in a plastic bag, ideally a special yellow biohazard bag, which should then be sealed and incinerated.

> **❶ WARNING**
> If you accidentally prick or cut your skin or splash your eyes, wash the area thoroughly and seek medical help immediately.

1

THIS CHAPTER outlines the core procedures that underpin first aid. Techniques for assessing a casualty are outlined first, followed by a guide to materials that make up a useful first-aid kit, and how to use them. Applying dressings and bandages is an essential part of first aid: wounds usually require a dressing, and most injuries benefit from the support of bandages.

CONTENTS

Monitoring vital signs.................8

First-aid materials....................10

Cold compresses.....................12

Sterile dressings 13

Principles of bandaging...........14

Triangular bandages...............16

Reef knots 16

Arm sling...............................17

Elevation sling........................18

TECHNIQUES AND EQUIPMENT

✦ FIRST-AID PRIORITIES

• Assess the casualty's condition.

• Comfort and reassure the casualty.

• Remove clothing if necessary.

• Use a first-aid technique relevant to the injury.

• Use dressings and bandages as needed.

• Monitor and record level of response, pulse, and breathing.

• Obtain medical aid if necessary. Call an ambulance at once if you suspect a serious illness or injury.

MONITORING VITAL SIGNS

When treating a casualty, you may need to assess and monitor his level of response, pulse, and breathing. You may also need to monitor temperature. These vital signs may help you to identify specific problems and indicate changes in a casualty's condition. Monitoring should be repeated regularly and your findings recorded on an observation chart (p.128), which should be handed to the medical assistance taking over.

CHECKING LEVEL OF RESPONSE

You will need to monitor a casualty's level of response in order to assess consciousness. Any injury or illness that affects the brain may affect consciousness, and any deterioration is potentially serious.

Assess the casualty's level of response using the AVPU code:
A – Is the casualty *Alert* ? Does the casualty open his eyes and respond to questions?

V – Does the casualty respond to *Voice*? Does he answer simple questions and obey commands?
P – Does the casualty respond to *Pain*? Does he open his eyes or move if he is pinched?
U – Is the casualty *Unresponsive* to any stimulus?

Using this code, you can check whether there is any change in the casualty's condition.

CHECKING PULSE

The normal pulse rate in adults is 60–80 beats per minute. The rate is faster in children and may be slower in very fit adults. An abnormally fast or slow pulse may be a sign of certain illnesses. The pulse may be measured at the neck (carotid pulse) or the wrist (radial pulse). In babies, the pulse in the upper arm (brachial pulse) may be easier to find.

When checking a pulse, use your fingers rather than your thumb (which has its own pulse), and press lightly until you can feel the pulse. Record the following points:
• Rate (the number of beats per minute).
• Strength (strong or weak).
• Rhythm (regular or irregular).

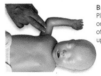

Brachial pulse
Place two fingers on the inner side of the infant's upper arm.

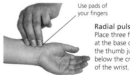

Use pads of your fingers

Radial pulse
Place three fingers at the base of the thumb just below the creases of the wrist.

Carotid pulse
Place two fingers on the side of the neck, in the hollow between the windpipe and the large neck muscle.

CHECKING BREATHING

When assessing a casualty's breathing, check the rate of breathing, listen for breathing difficulties or noises, and watch the casualty's chest movements. The normal breathing rate in adults is 12–16 breaths per minute; in babies and young children it is 20–30 breaths per minute. For a baby or young child, place your hand on the chest and feel for breathing. Record the following:

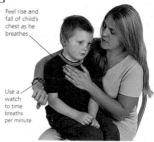
Feel rise and fall of child's chest as he breathes

Use a watch to time breaths per minute

- Rate (number of breaths per minute).
- Depth (deep or shallow breaths).
- Ease (whether breaths are easy, difficult, or painful).
- Noise (whether breathing is quiet or noisy, and types of noise).

Assessing breathing rate
Watch the chest move and count the number of breaths per minute. For a baby or young child, it may be easier if you place your hand on the chest.

CHECKING TEMPERATURE

To assess body temperature, you need to feel exposed skin and obtain an accurate reading using a thermometer. Normal body temperature is 37°C (98.6°F). A high temperature (fever) is usually caused by infection. A low body temperature (hypothermia) may result from exposure to cold and/or wet conditions. There are several types of thermometer, including traditional glass mercury and digital models, so ensure that you know how to use them.

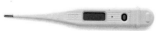

Digital thermometer
This can be used to measure temperature under the tongue or under the armpit. Leave it in place until it makes a beeping sound (about 30 seconds), then read the temperature from the display.

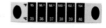

Forehead thermometer
This heat-sensitive strip is useful for measuring temperature in a young child. Hold the strip against the child's forehead for about 30 seconds. A change in colour on the strip indicates the temperature.

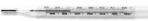

Mercury thermometer
Before using this thermometer check that the mercury level is below 37°C (98.6°F). Leave the thermometer in position (under the tongue or in the armpit) for 2–3 minutes before reading.

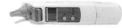

Ear sensor
The tip of this thermometer is placed inside the ear and gives a reading within 1 second. The sensor is easy to use and is especially useful for a sick child. It can be used while the child is asleep.

FIRST-AID MATERIALS

All workplaces, leisure centres, homes, and cars should have first-aid kits. The kits for workplaces or leisure centres must conform to legal requirements; they should also be clearly marked and easily accessible. For a home or a car, you can either buy a kit or assemble first-aid items yourself and keep them in a clean, waterproof container. Any first-aid kit must be kept in a dry place, and checked and replenished regularly.

The items on these pages (see also p.12) form the basis of a home first-aid kit. You may wish to add items such as aspirin and paracetamol.

DRESSINGS

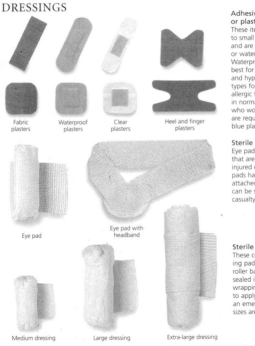

Fabric plasters

Waterproof plasters

Clear plasters

Heel and finger plasters

Eye pad

Eye pad with headband

Medium dressing

Large dressing

Extra-large dressing

Adhesive dressings or plasters
These items are applied to small cuts and grazes and are made of fabric or waterproof plastic. Waterproof types are best for hand wounds, and hypoallergenic types for anyone who is allergic to the adhesive in normal ones. People who work with food are required to use blue plasters.

Sterile eye pads
Eye pads are dressings that are used to protect injured eyes. Some eye pads have bandages attached so that they can be secured to a casualty's head.

Sterile dressings
These consist of a dressing pad attached to a roller bandage, and are sealed in a protective wrapping. They are easy to apply, so are ideal in an emergency. Various sizes are available.

BANDAGES

Self-adhesive
roller bandage

Crêpe roller
bandage

Open-weave roller
bandage

Roller bandages
These items are used to give support to injured joints, restrict movement, secure dressings in place and maintain pressure on them, and limit swelling.

Elasticated roller
bandage

Conforming roller
bandage

Crêpe conforming
roller bandage

Folded cloth
triangular bandage

Folded paper
triangular bandage

Triangular bandages
Made of cloth or strong paper, these items can be used as bandages and slings. If they are sterile and individually wrapped, they may also be used as dressings for large wounds and burns.

BASIC MATERIALS FOR A HOME FIRST-AID KIT

- Easily identifiable watertight box.
- 20 adhesive dressings (plasters) in assorted sizes.
- Two crêpe roller bandages.
- Six medium sterile dressings.
- Two large sterile dressings.
- Two extra-large sterile dressings.
- Two sterile eye pads.
- Six triangular bandages.
- Six safety pins.
- Disposable gloves.

Useful additions:
- Scissors.
- Tweezers.
- Cotton wool.
- Non-alcoholic wound cleansing wipes.
- Adhesive tape.
- Plastic face shield or pocket face mask.
- Notepad, pencil, and tags.
- Blanket, survival bag, torch, whistle.

FIRST-AID MATERIALS (continued)

ADDITIONAL ITEMS FOR A HOME FIRST-AID KIT

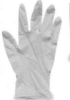

Gauze pads
Use these as dressings, as padding, or as swabs to clean around wounds.

Cleansing wipes
Alcohol-free wipes can be used to clean skin around wounds, or to clean your hands if water and soap are not available.

Disposable gloves
Wear gloves, if available, whenever you dress wounds or when you handle body fluids or other waste materials.

Face protection
Use a plastic face shield (left) or a pocket mask (right) to protect you and the casualty from infections when giving rescue breaths.

Bandage clip

Safety pins

Pins and clips
These items can be used to secure the ends of bandages.

COLD COMPRESSES

Cooling an injury such as a bruise or sprain can reduce swelling and pain, although it will not relieve the injury itself. There are two types of compress: cold pads, which are made from material dampened with cold water; and ice packs, which are cold items (such as ice cubes or packs of frozen peas or other vegetables) wrapped in a dry cloth.

COLD PAD

1 Soak a flannel or towel in very cold water. Wring it out lightly, fold it into a pad, then place it firmly on the injury.

2 Re-soak the pad in cold water every 3–5 minutes to keep it cold. Cool the injury for at least 10 minutes.

ICE PACK

1 Partly fill a plastic bag with small ice cubes or crushed ice, or use a pack of frozen vegetables. Wrap the bag in a dry cloth.

> **❶ CAUTION**
>
> To prevent cold injuries, always wrap an ice pack in a cloth; and do not use it for more than 10 minutes at one application.

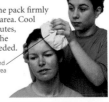

2 Hold the pack firmly on the area. Cool for 10 minutes, replacing the pack as needed.

Cover injury and surrounding area with pack

STERILE DRESSINGS

This type of dressing consists of a dressing pad attached to a roller bandage. The pad consists of gauze backed by a layer of cotton wool.

Sterile dressings are sold individually in various sizes and they are sealed in protective wrappings to prevent contamination. Once the seal on this type of dressing has been broken, the dressing is no longer sterile.

> **⚠ CAUTION**
>
> • If the dressing slips out of place, remove it and apply a new dressing.
> • If bleeding appears through the dressing, apply another on top of the original one. If blood seeps through the second dressing as well, take off both dressings and apply a fresh dressing.
> • Take care not to impair the circulation beyond the dressing.

1 Break the seal and remove the wrapping. Unwind the bandage, taking care not to drop the roll or touch the dressing pad.

2 Unfold the dressing pad, holding the bandage on each side of it. Lay the pad directly on the wound.

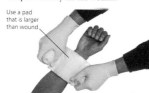

Use a pad that is larger than wound

3 Wind the short end (tail) of the bandage once around the limb and the dressing to secure the pad.

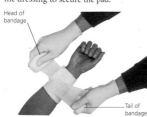

Head of bandage

Tail of bandage

4 Wind the other end (head) of the bandage around the limb to cover the whole pad. Leave the tail of the bandage hanging free.

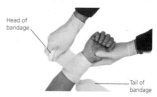

Head of bandage

Tail of bandage

5 To secure the bandage, tie the ends in a reef knot (p.16). Tie the knot directly over the pad to exert firm pressure on the wound.

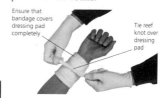

Ensure that bandage covers dressing pad completely

Tie reef knot over dressing pad

6 Once you have secured the bandage, check the circulation in the limb beyond it (p.14). Loosen the bandage if it is too tight.

PRINCIPLES OF BANDAGING

There are a number of different first-aid uses for bandages: they can be used to secure dressings, control bleeding, support and immobilise limbs, and reduce swelling in an injured part. If you have no bandage available, you can improvise one from an everyday item; for example, you can fold a square of fabric, such as a headscarf, diagonally to make a triangular bandage (p.16).

⊙ See also ROLLER BANDAGES opposite
▪ TRIANGULAR BANDAGES p.16

RULES FOR APPLYING A BANDAGE

• Make the casualty comfortable, in a suitable sitting or lying position and explain what you are going to do.
• Keep the injured part supported while you are working on it. Ask the casualty or a helper to do this.
• Work at the front of the casualty, and from the injured side if possible.
• If the casualty is lying down, pass the bandages under hollows at the ankles, knees, waist, and neck, then slide the bandages back and forth under the body into position.
• Leave the fingers or toes on a bandaged limb exposed, if possible, so that you can check the circulation.
• Tie bandages with reef knots (p.16).
• Regularly check the circulation in the area beyond the bandage (below). If necessary, unroll the bandage until the blood supply returns, and reapply it more loosely.

CHECKING CIRCULATION AFTER BANDAGING

When bandaging a limb or using a sling, check the circulation in the hand or foot immediately after you have finished bandaging, and every 10 minutes thereafter. These checks are essential because limbs swell after an injury, and a bandage can rapidly become too tight and interfere with blood circulation to the area beyond it. Symptoms of impaired circulation change as first the veins and then the arteries become constricted.

> **RECOGNITION**
>
> *If circulation is impaired there may be:*
> • A swollen and congested limb.
> • Blue skin with prominent veins.
> • A feeling that the skin is painfully distended.
> *Later there may be:*
> • Pale, waxy skin.
> • Cold numbness.
> • Tingling, followed by deep pain.
> • Inability to move affected fingers or toes.

1 Briefly press one of the nails, or the skin, until it turns pale, then release the pressure. If the colour does not return, or returns slowly, the bandage may be too tight.

2 Loosen a tight bandage by unrolling just enough turns for warmth and colour to return to the skin. The casualty may feel a tingling sensation. Reapply the bandage.

APPLYING A ROLLER BANDAGE

Follow these general rules when you are applying a roller bandage:

- Keep the rolled part of the bandage (the "head") uppermost as you work (the unrolled part is called the "tail").
- Position yourself towards the front of the casualty, on the injured side.
- Make sure that the injured part is supported in the position in which it will remain after bandaging.

> **❶ CAUTION**
>
> Once you have applied the bandage, check the circulation in the limb beyond it (opposite). This is especially important if you are applying an elasticated or crepe bandage because these mould to the shape of the limb and may become tighter if the limb swells.

1 Place the tail of the bandage below the injury. Bandaging from the inside of the limb outwards, make two straight turns to anchor the tail in place.

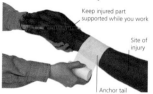

Keep injured part supported while you work

Site of injury

Anchor tail

2 Make a series of spiralling turns with the bandage. Wind it from the inside to the outside of the upper surface of the limb, working upwards. Each new turn should cover between one half and two-thirds of the previous turn of bandaging.

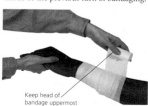

Keep head of bandage uppermost

3 Finish with one straight turn, and secure the end of the bandage. If the bandage is too short, apply another one so that the injured area is covered.

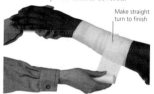

Make straight turn to finish

4 As soon as you have finished, check the circulation beyond the bandage (opposite). If necessary, unroll the bandage until the blood supply returns, and reapply it more loosely.

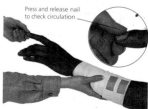

Press and release nail to check circulation

TRIANGULAR BANDAGES

This type of bandage may be supplied as part of a first-aid kit. To make one, cut or fold a square metre of sturdy fabric diagonally in half. The bandage can be used in the following ways:

● Folded into a broad-fold bandage (below) to immobilise and support a limb or to secure a splint or dressing.
● Folded into a narrow-fold bandage (below) to immobilise feet and ankles or hold a dressing in place.
● Opened to form a sling.

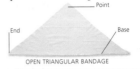

OPEN TRIANGULAR BANDAGE

MAKING A BROAD-FOLD BANDAGE

1 Open a triangular bandage and lay it flat on a clean surface. Fold it in half horizontally, so that the point of the triangle touches the centre of the base.

2 Fold the triangular bandage in half again, in the same direction, so that the first folded edge touches the base. The bandage should now form a broad strip.

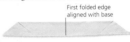

End | Point | Base

First folded edge aligned with base

MAKING A NARROW-FOLD BANDAGE

1 Fold a triangular bandage to make a broad-fold bandage (above).

2 Fold the bandage horizontally in half again. It should form a long, narrow strip of material.

REEF KNOTS

Always use a reef knot to secure a triangular bandage. It will not slip; it is easy to untie; and it lies flat, so it is more comfortable for the casualty. Avoid tying the knot around or directly over the injury itself.

TYING A REEF KNOT

1 Pass the left end (dark) over and under the right end (light).

2 Lift both ends of the bandage above the rest of the material.

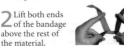

3 Pass the right end (dark) over and under the left end (light).

4 Pull the ends to tighten the knot, then tuck them under the bandage.

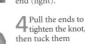

ARM SLING

An arm sling holds the forearm in a horizontal or slightly raised position. It provides support for an injured upper arm, wrist, or forearm, and is used for a casualty whose elbow can be bent. An elevation sling (p.18) is used to keep the forearm and hand raised in a higher position.

1 Make sure that the injured arm is supported with its hand slightly raised. Fold the base of the bandage under to form a hem. Place the bandage with the base parallel to the casualty's body and level with her little finger nail. Pass the upper end under the injured arm and then pull it around the neck to the opposite shoulder.

3 Tie a reef knot (opposite) on the injured side, at the hollow above the casualty's collar bone. Tuck both free ends of the bandage under the knot to pad it.

Tie knot just above collar bone

Ensure sling supports forearm and hand up to little finger

4 Fold the point forwards at the casualty's elbow. Tuck loose fabric around the elbow, and secure the point to the front with a safety pin. If you do not have a pin, twist the point until the fabric fits the elbow snugly, then tuck it into the sling at the back of the arm.

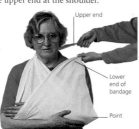

Pass end over shoulder and around back of neck

Hold point beyond elbow

2 Fold the lower end of the bandage up over the forearm and bring it to meet the upper end at the shoulder.

Upper end

Lower end of bandage

Point

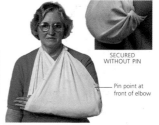

SECURED WITHOUT PIN

Pin point at front of elbow

5 As soon as you have finished, check the circulation in the fingers (p.14). Recheck every 10 minutes. If necessary, loosen and reapply the bandages and sling.

ELEVATION SLING

This type of sling supports the forearm and hand in a raised position, with the fingertips touching the casualty's shoulder. The elevation sling helps to control bleeding from wounds in the forearm or hand, minimise swelling in burn injuries, and support the chest in complicated rib fractures.

1 Ask the casualty to support his injured arm across his chest, with the fingers resting on the opposite shoulder.

Ask casualty to support his elbow

2 Place the bandage over his body, with one end over the uninjured shoulder. Hold the point just beyond his elbow.

Base of bandage

Hold point beyond elbow of injured side

3 Ask the casualty to let go of his injured arm. Tuck the base of the bandage under his hand, forearm, and elbow.

Support arm as you work

Leave thumb showing

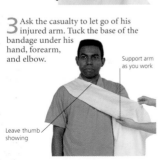

4 Bring the lower end of the bandage up diagonally across his back, to meet the other end at his shoulder.

Bring ends together

Pass lower end of bandage up across back

5 Tie the ends in a reef knot (p.16) at the hollow above the casualty's collar bone. Tuck the ends under the knot so that they pad it.

6 Twist the point until the bandage fits closely around the casualty's elbow. Tuck the point in just above his elbow to secure it. If you have a safety pin, fold the fabric over the elbow, and fasten the point at the corner.

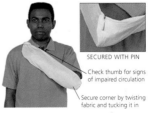

SECURED WITH PIN

Check thumb for signs of impaired circulation

Secure corner by twisting fabric and tucking it in

7 Regularly check the circulation in the thumb (p.14). If necessary, loosen and reapply the bandages and sling.

2

TO STAY ALIVE we need an adequate supply of oxygen to enter the lungs and be transferred to all cells in the body through the bloodstream. If a casualty is deprived of oxygen, the brain begins to fail. The casualty will lose consciousness, the heartbeat and breathing will cease, and death results.

RESUSCITATION

To restore oxygen to the brain, the airway must be open so that oxygen can enter the body; breathing must be restored to enable oxygen to enter the bloodstream via the lungs; and blood must circulate to all tissues and organs. Therefore, the priority in treating any collapsed casualty is to establish an open airway and maintain breathing and circulation. Because treatment differs for children and infants, this chapter gives separate step-by-step instructions for adults, children, and infants. Techniques for treating an adult, child, or infant who is choking are also given in this chapter.

✚ FIRST-AID PRIORITIES

• Maintain an open airway, check breathing, and resuscitate.
• If casualty is choking, relieve airway obstruction if possible.

CONTENTS

Life-saving priorities 20

Adult resuscitation chart 21

Unconscious adult....................22

Child resuscitation chart...........32

Unconscious child
    (1–7 years)...................33

Infant resuscitation chart.........40

Unconscious infant
    (under 1 year)...............41

Choking summary charts 45

Choking adult..........................46

Choking child
    (1–7 years).......................47

Choking infant
    (under 1 year)...................48

LIFE-SAVING PROCEDURES

LIFE-SAVING PRIORITIES

With an unconscious casualty, your priorities are:

● *To maintain an open airway*. In an unconscious casualty, muscular control may be lost, so the tongue may fall back and block the airway. Lifting the chin and tilting the head back lifts the tongue from the entrance to the air passage, so allowing the casualty to breathe.

● *To breathe for the casualty*. By giving rescue breaths you can force air into the casualty's air passages and so get oxygen into the bloodstream and circulating around the body.

● *To maintain blood circulation*. Chest compressions can be used to artificially maintain blood circulation and so get oxygen-rich blood to the tissues. To make sure that the blood is adequately supplied with oxygen, chest compressions must always be combined with rescue breathing (together known as cardiopulmonary resuscitation or CPR).

In addition, a machine called a defibrillator can deliver a controlled electric shock that can restore a normal heartbeat.

The following factors increase the chances of survival if all elements are complete:

● Help is called quickly.
● Blood circulation is maintained by CPR.
● In an adult casualty with no signs of circulation, a defibrillator is used promptly.
● The casualty reaches hospital quickly for specialised treatment.

Chain of survival
Four elements increase the chances of a collapsed adult casualty surviving. If any one of the elements in this chain is missing, the chances are reduced.

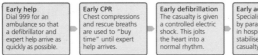

Early help	Early CPR	Early defibrillation	Early advanced care
Dial 999 for an ambulance so that a defibrillator and expert help arrive as quickly as possible.	Chest compressions and rescue breaths are used to "buy time" until expert help arrives.	The casualty is given a controlled electric shock. This jolts the heart into a normal rhythm.	Specialised treatment by paramedics and in hospital quickly stabilises the casualty's condition.

WHEN TO CALL AN AMBULANCE

If you have a helper, send him to call for an ambulance as soon as you know that the casualty is not breathing. If you are on your own, your actions depend on the age of the casualty and likely cause of the unconsciousness.

CHILD OR INFANT CASUALTY
Unconsciousness in an infant or child under 8 years is most likely to be due to a breathing problem. For this reason, you should give rescue breaths and chest compressions for 1 minute before leaving the child to call an ambulance.

ADULT CASUALTY
If an adult casualty's unconsciousness is due to a heart problem, or the cause is unknown, call for an ambulance immediately if breathing is absent. If unconsciousness is due to injury, drowning, or choking, give chest compressions and rescue breaths for 1 minute, then call an ambulance.

ADULT RESUSCITATION CHART

The sequence below summarises the main actions for dealing with an adult, or child aged 8 or over, who is unconscious. The chart assumes that you have checked for any danger to yourself or the casualty. The pages that follow give full details on each step in the resuscitation sequence.

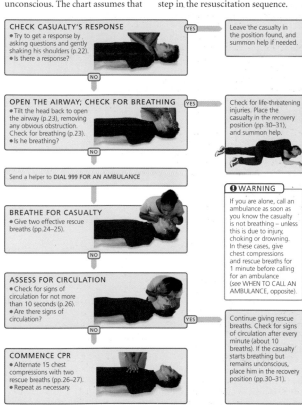

CHECK CASUALTY'S RESPONSE
- Try to get a response by asking questions and gently shaking his shoulders (p.22).
- Is there a response?

YES → Leave the casualty in the position found, and summon help if needed.

NO

OPEN THE AIRWAY; CHECK FOR BREATHING
- Tilt the head back to open the airway (p.23), removing any obvious obstruction. Check for breathing (p.23).
- Is he breathing?

YES → Check for life-threatening injuries. Place the casualty in the recovery position (pp 30–31), and summon help.

NO

Send a helper to **DIAL 999 FOR AN AMBULANCE**

BREATHE FOR CASUALTY
- Give two effective rescue breaths (pp.24–25).

NO

ASSESS FOR CIRCULATION
- Check for signs of circulation for not more than 10 seconds (p.26).
- Are there signs of circulation?

YES →

NO

COMMENCE CPR
- Alternate 15 chest compressions with two rescue breaths (pp.26–27).
- Repeat as necessary.

! WARNING

If you are alone, call an ambulance as soon as you know the casualty is not breathing – unless this is due to injury, choking or drowning. In these cases, give chest compressions and rescue breaths for 1 minute before calling for an ambulance (*see* WHEN TO CALL AN AMBULANCE, opposite).

Continue giving rescue breaths. Check for signs of circulation after every minute (about 10 breaths). If the casualty starts breathing but remains unconscious, place him in the recovery position (pp.30–31).

21

UNCONSCIOUS ADULT

The following pages give instructions for all the techniques needed in the resuscitation of an unconscious adult.

Always approach the casualty from the side, kneeling next to his head or chest. You will then be in the correct position for all the possible stages of resuscitation: opening the casualty's airway; checking breathing and circulation; and giving rescue breaths and chest compressions (called CPR or cardiopulmonary resuscitation).

At each stage, you will have decisions to make. The steps given here tell you what to do next in each situation.

The first priority is to open the airway so the casualty can breathe or you can give effective rescue breaths. If breathing and circulation return at any stage, place the casualty in the recovery position. If there is no breathing or signs of circulation, a defibrillator, correctly used, increases the chance of survival.

HOW TO CHECK RESPONSE

On discovering a collapsed casualty, you should first establish whether he is conscious or unconscious. Do this by gently shaking the casualty's shoulders. Ask "What has happened?" or give a command: "Open your eyes". Speak loudly and clearly.

> **❶ CAUTION**
>
> Always assume that there is a neck injury and shake the shoulders very gently.

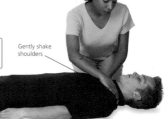

Gently shake shoulders

IF THERE IS A RESPONSE

1 If there is no further danger, leave the casualty in the position in which he was found and summon help if needed.

2 Treat any condition found and monitor vital signs – level of response, pulse, and breathing (pp.8–9).

3 Continue monitoring the casualty until either help arrives or he recovers.

IF THERE IS NO RESPONSE

1 Shout for help. If possible, leave the casualty in the position in which he was found and open the airway.

2 If this is not possible, turn him onto his back and open the airway.

▶ Go to HOW TO OPEN THE AIRWAY opposite

HOW TO OPEN THE AIRWAY

1 Kneel by the casualty's head. Place one hand on his forehead. Gently tilt his head back. The mouth will fall open.

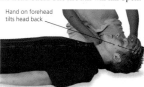

Hand on forehead tilts head back

3 Place the fingertips of your other hand under the point of the casualty's chin and lift the chin.

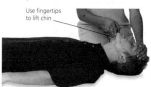

Use fingertips to lift chin

2 Pick out any obvious obstructions, such as dislodged dentures or broken teeth, from the casualty's mouth. Do not do a finger sweep. Leave well-fitting dentures in place.

4 Check to see if the casualty is now breathing.

▶ Go to HOW TO CHECK BREATHING below

HOW TO CHECK BREATHING

Keeping the airway open, look, listen, and feel for breathing: look for chest movement, listen for sounds of breathing, and feel for breath on your cheek. Wait no more than 10 seconds before deciding breathing is absent.

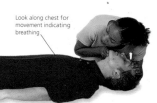

Look along chest for movement indicating breathing

IF CASUALTY IS BREATHING

1 Check the casualty for any life-threatening injuries, such as severe bleeding, and treat as necessary.

2 Place the casualty in the recovery position. Monitor vital signs – response, pulse, and breathing (pp.8–9).

▶ Go to HOW TO PLACE IN RECOVERY POSITION pp.30–31

IF CASUALTY IS NOT BREATHING

1 DIAL 999 FOR AN AMBULANCE Send a helper if available. If you are alone, *see* WHEN TO CALL AN AMBULANCE, p.20.

2 Give two effective rescue breaths and then check for signs of circulation.

▶ Go to HOW TO GIVE RESCUE BREATHS pp.24–25

UNCONSCIOUS ADULT (continued)

HOW TO GIVE RESCUE BREATHS

1 Make sure that the casualty's airway is still open, by keeping one hand on his forehead and two fingers of the other hand under the tip of his chin.

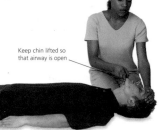

Keep chin lifted so that airway is open

2 Move the hand that was on the forehead down to the nose. Pinch the soft part of the nose with the finger and thumb. Open the casualty's mouth.

3 If you have a face shield or pocket mask (below), place it over the casualty's mouth. Take a deep breath to fill your lungs with air and place your lips around the casualty's mouth, making sure you have a good seal.

Continue to pinch the nose while taking a breath

SPECIAL CASE

USING A FACE SHIELD OR POCKET MASK
First aiders may receive training in the use of these hygiene aids. Face shields are plastic barriers with a reinforced hole to fit over the casualty's mouth. The mask is more substantial and has a valve.

If you are trained to use one of these aids, carry it with you at all times and use it if you need to resuscitate a casualty. If you do not have a mask or shield, do not hesitate to give rescue breaths.

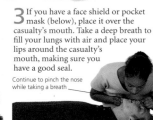

USING A FACE SHIELD   USING A POCKET MASK

4 Blow steadily into the casualty's mouth until the chest rises. This usually takes about 2 seconds.

5 Maintaining head tilt and chin lift, remove your mouth and see if the casualty's chest falls. If it rises visibly as you blow and falls fully when you lift your mouth away, you have given an effective breath. Give two effective breaths, then check for circulation.

▶ Go to HOW TO CHECK FOR CIRCULATION p.26

Watch the chest fall

IF YOU CANNOT ACHIEVE EFFECTIVE BREATHS

• Recheck the head tilt and chin lift.
• Recheck the casualty's mouth. Remove any obvious obstructions, but do not do a finger sweep of the mouth.
• Make no more than five attempts to achieve two effective breaths.

If you still cannot achieve two effective breaths, check the casualty for signs of circulation.

▶ Go to HOW TO CHECK FOR CIRCULATION p.26

❶ **WARNING**

If you know that the casualty has choked, and you cannot achieve effective breaths, you must immediately begin giving chest compressions and rescue breaths to try to relieve the obstruction quickly (see HOW TO GIVE CPR, pp.26–27).

SPECIAL CASE

MOUTH-TO-NOSE RESCUE BREATHING
In situations such as rescue from water, or where injuries to the mouth make it impossible to achieve a good seal, use the mouth-to-nose method for giving rescue breaths. With the casualty's mouth closed, form a tight seal with your lips around the nose and blow steadily into the casualty's nose. Then allow the mouth to fall open to let the air escape.

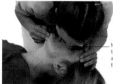

Make a tight seal around the nose

SPECIAL CASE

MOUTH-TO-STOMA RESCUE BREATHING
A casualty who has had the voice-box surgically removed breathes through a stoma (opening) in the front of the neck rather than the mouth and nose. Always check for a stoma before giving rescue breaths. If you find a stoma, close off the mouth and nose with your thumb and fingers and then breathe into the stoma.

Close off casualty's mouth and nose with your thumb and fingers

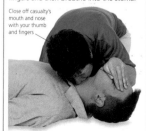

UNCONSCIOUS ADULT (continued)

HOW TO CHECK FOR CIRCULATION

Still kneeling beside the casualty's head, look, listen, and feel for signs of circulation, such as breathing, coughing, or movement. Carry out this check for no more than 10 seconds.

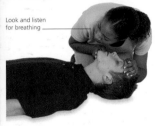

Look and listen for breathing

IF THERE ARE NO SIGNS OF CIRCULATION
Begin giving chest compressions with rescue breaths immediately.

▶ Go to HOW TO GIVE CPR below

IF YOU ARE SURE YOU HAVE DETECTED SIGNS OF CIRCULATION

1 Continue rescue breathing. After every 10 breaths (about 1 minute), recheck for signs of circulation. If the casualty starts to breathe but remains unconscious, turn him into the recovery position (pp.30–31).

2 Monitor vital signs – level of response, pulse, and breathing (pp.8–9). Be prepared to turn the casualty on to his back again to restart rescue breathing (pp.24–25).

HOW TO GIVE CPR

1 Kneel beside the casualty. With the index and middle fingers of your lower hand, locate one of his lowermost ribs on the side nearest to you. Slide your fingertips along the rib to the point where the lowermost ribs meet at the breastbone. Place your middle finger at this point and your index finger beside it on the lower breastbone.

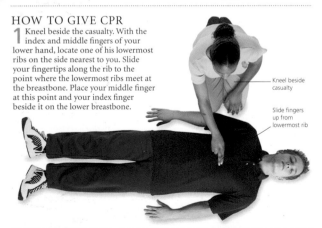

Kneel beside casualty

Slide fingers up from lowermost rib

2 Place the heel of your other hand on the breastbone, and slide it down until it reaches your index finger. This is the point at which you should apply pressure.

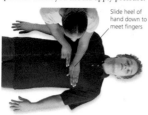

Slide heel of hand down to meet fingers

3 Place the heel of your first hand on top of the other hand, and interlock your fingers.

Keep fingers clear of chest

4 Leaning well over the casualty, with your arms straight, press down vertically on the breastbone and depress the chest by about 4–5 cm (1½–2 in). Release the pressure without removing your hands from his chest.

5 Compress the chest 15 times at a rate of 100 compressions per minute. The time taken for compression and release should be about the same.

6 Tilt the head, lift the chin, and give two rescue breaths (pp.24–25).

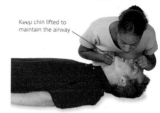

Keep chin lifted to maintain the airway

7 Continue this cycle of alternating 15 chest compressions with two rescue breaths. Continue with CPR until emergency help arrives and takes over; the casualty makes a movement or takes a spontaneous breath; or you become so exhausted that you cannot carry on.

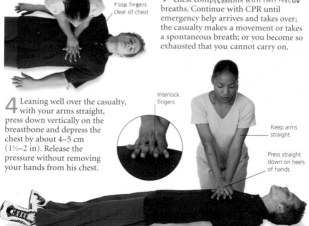

Interlock fingers

Keep arms straight

Press straight down on heels of hands

UNCONSCIOUS ADULT (continued)

HOW TO USE A DEFIBRILLATOR

When the heart stops and there are no signs of circulation, a cardiac arrest has occurred. The most common cause is an abnormal heart rhythm, known as ventricular fibrillation. This can be caused by a heart attack or when the heart has insufficient oxygen. The rhythm can be corrected with a defibrillator (automated external defibrillator, or AED). These are available in many public places, including airports, some shopping centres, and railway stations. A defibrillator analyses the casualty's heart rhythm and tells you what action to take at each stage. However, you must be trained in its use and be able to carry out CPR (pp.26–27).

You will probably have already started the life-saving sequence when the defibrillator arrives. Stop what you are doing and start using it.

> **⊘ CAUTION**
>
> • Make sure that no-one is touching the casualty because this will interfere with the defibrillator readings.
>
> • Do not turn off the defibrillator or remove the pads at any point, even if the casualty appears to have recovered.

1 Switch on the defibrillator and check that the electrode leads are plugged in. Remove or cut through clothing covering the chest and quickly wipe away any sweat. Shave chest hair if it is excessive because it will prevent the pads from sticking to the skin.

2 Remove the backing paper from the electrode pads and attach them to the casualty's chest in the position indicated on the pads.

3 The defibrillator will start analysing the heart rhythm: ensure no-one is touching the casualty. Follow the visual and/or spoken prompts (opposite). These will advise you when a shock is indicated, when to check for signs of circulation (p.26), and when to give chest compressions and rescue breaths (see HOW TO GIVE CPR, pp.26–27).

4 Continue to follow the prompts from the defibrillator until the emergency services arrive and advanced care is available. If at any time the casualty starts breathing, place him in the recovery position (pp.30–31). Leave the defibrillator attached.

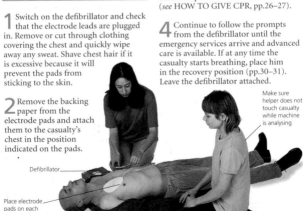

Make sure helper does not touch casualty while machine is analysing

Defibrillator

Place electrode pads on each side of heart

SEQUENCE OF DEFIBRILLATOR INSTRUCTIONS

The defibrillator will give a series of visual and verbal prompts as soon as it is switched on. Some older machines may tell you to check the pulse. In this case, you must in fact check for circulation. Do not waste time trying to find the pulse. Continue to follow the prompts given by the defibrillator until the emergency services arrive and advanced care is available.

> • Switch defibrillator on and make sure leads are connected.
> • Attach pads to casualty's chest.

> Defibrillator gets ready to analyse the casualty's heart. It may state "Stand clear, analysing now" or just "Analysing". Make sure no-one is touching the casualty or the defibrillator will be unable to analyse. Is shock advised?

YES / NO

YES:

> Defibrillator advises that a shock is needed. The machine charges up; an alarm sounds when the machine is ready.

> Defibrillator instructs you to deliver the shock.
> • Make sure everyone is clear of the casualty.
> • Push the shock button.
> Defibrillator delivers the shock and then re-analyses the heart rhythm. You may be prompted to give up to three shocks.

> Defibrillator instructs you to check for circulation (older machines may state "check pulse" – always check circulation).
> • Check for signs of circulation (p.26) for no more than 10 seconds. Is there circulation?

YES / NO

> • Check airway and breathing (p.23).

> • Start CPR (pp.26–27) as instructed. Continue for 1 minute (until machine prompts you to stop).

> The defibrillator re-analyses heart rhythm.

NO:

> Defibrillator advises that no shock is needed.

> Defibrillator instructs you to check for circulation (older machines may state "check pulse" – always check circulation).
> • Look for signs of circulation (p.26) for no more than 10 seconds. Is there circulation?

YES / NO

> • Check airway and breathing (p.23).

> • Start CPR (pp.26–27). Continue for 1 minute (until machine prompts you to stop).

> The defibrillator re-analyses heart rhythm.

UNCONSCIOUS ADULT (continued)

HOW TO PLACE IN RECOVERY POSITION

1 Kneel beside the casualty. Remove spectacles and any very bulky objects, such as mobile phones and large bunches of keys, from the pockets. Do not search the pockets for small items.

2 Make sure that both of the casualty's legs are straight.

3 Place the arm that is nearest to you at right angles to the casualty's body, with the elbow bent and the palm of the hand facing upwards.

⊙ WARNING

If you suspect a spinal injury, and you cannot maintain an open airway with the casualty in the position in which he was found, or by using the jaw thrust method (p.81), use the guidelines opposite for turning him.

⊙ CAUTION

If the casualty is found lying on his side or front, not all these steps will be necessary to place him in the recovery position.

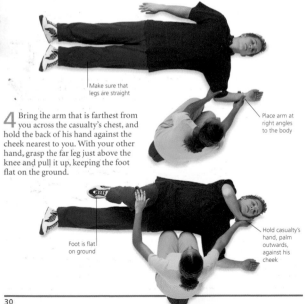

Make sure that legs are straight

Place arm at right angles to the body

4 Bring the arm that is farthest from you across the casualty's chest, and hold the back of his hand against the cheek nearest to you. With your other hand, grasp the far leg just above the knee and pull it up, keeping the foot flat on the ground.

Foot is flat on ground

Hold casualty's hand, palm outwards, against his cheek

5 Keeping the casualty's hand pressed against his cheek, pull on the far leg and roll the casualty towards you and on to his side.

Hold on to casualty's leg and pull it over

6 Adjust the upper leg so that both the hip and the knee are bent at right angles.

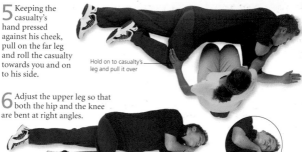

Bent leg props up body and prevents casualty from rolling forwards

Hand under cheek helps to keep airway open

8 If it has not already been done, **DIAL 999 FOR AN AMBULANCE** Monitor and record vital signs – level of response, pulse, and breathing (pp.8–9).

7 Tilt the casualty's head back so that the airway remains open. If necessary, adjust the hand under the cheek to make sure that the head remains tilted and the airway stays open.

9 If the casualty has to be left in the recovery position for longer than 30 minutes, roll him on to his back, and then turn him on to the opposite side – unless other injuries prevent this.

SPECIAL CASE

SPINAL INJURY
If you suspect a spinal injury and need to place the casualty in the recovery position to maintain an open airway, it is important to try to keep the spine straight using the following guidelines:

• If you are alone, use the technique shown on this page.

• If you have a helper, one of you should steady the head while the other turns the casualty (right).

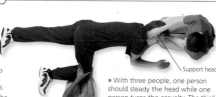

Support head

Helper puts casualty into position

• With three people, one person should steady the head while one person turns the casualty. The third person should keep the casualty's back straight during the manoeuvre.

• If there are four or more people in total available to help, use the log-roll technique (p.81).

CHILD RESUSCITATION CHART

The resuscitation method depends on the child's age and size. In children aged 1–7, respiratory failure (absence of breathing) is the main reason for the heart to stop. Ask a helper to call an ambulance while you treat the child; if you are alone, resuscitate for 1 minute before calling an ambulance.

For a child aged 8 or over, use adult resuscitation methods (pp.21–31).

CHECK CHILD'S RESPONSE
- Try to get a response by asking questions and gently tapping the child's shoulder.
- Is there a response?

YES → Leave the child in the position found and summon help if needed.

NO ↓

OPEN THE AIRWAY; CHECK FOR BREATHING
- Tilt the head back to open the airway (p.34), removing any obvious obstruction. Check for breathing (p.34).
- Is the child breathing?

YES → Check for life-threatening injuries. Place the child in the recovery position (pp.38–39) and summon help.

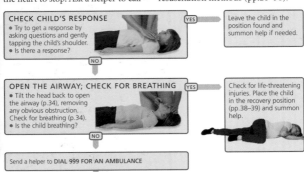

NO ↓

Send a helper to **DIAL 999 FOR AN AMBULANCE**

BREATHE FOR CHILD
- Give two effective rescue breaths (p.35).

NO ↓

> **❶ WARNING**
>
> If you are alone, carry out rescue breathing and chest compressions for 1 minute before leaving the child to call for help (see WHEN TO CALL AN AMBULANCE, p.20).

ASSESS FOR CIRCULATION
- Check for circulation for no more than 10 seconds (p.36).
- Are there signs of circulation?

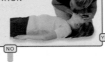

YES → Continue rescue breathing. After every 20 breaths (about 1 minute), recheck for signs of circulation. If the child starts to breathe but remains unconscious, place her in the recovery position (pp.38–39).

NO ↓

COMMENCE CPR
- Alternate five chest compressions with one rescue breath (pp.36–37).
- Repeat as necessary.

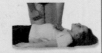

UNCONSCIOUS CHILD (1–7 years)

The following pages give instructions for resuscitating a child aged 1–7 who collapses. For a child aged 8 or over, use the adult method (pp.21–31).

Always approach the child from the side, kneeling next to the head or chest. You will then be in the correct position for all the possible stages of resuscitation: opening the airway, checking the breathing and circulation, and giving rescue breaths and chest compressions (called CPR or cardiopulmonary resuscitation).

The steps given here will guide you through each technique, then advise you on what to do next. Your first priority is to ensure that the airway is clear so that the child can breathe or you can give effective rescue breaths if needed. If normal breathing and circulation resume, place the child in the recovery position (pp.38–39).

Call an ambulance immediately if a child who has a known heart disease collapses because early access to advanced care may be life-saving.

HOW TO CHECK FOR RESPONSE

On discovering a collapsed child, you should first establish whether she is conscious or unconscious. Do this by speaking loudly and clearly to the child. Ask "What has happened?" or give a command: "Open your eyes". Place one hand on her shoulder, and gently tap her.

Gently tap shoulder

IF THERE IS A RESPONSE

1 If there is no further danger, leave the child in the position in which she was found and summon help if needed.

2 Treat any condition found. Regularly monitor vital signs – level of response, pulse, and breathing (pp.8–9).

3 Continue this until either help arrives or the child recovers.

IF THERE IS NO RESPONSE

1 Shout for help. If possible, leave the child in the position in which she was found, then open the airway.

2 If this is not possible, turn the child on to her back and open the airway.

▶ Go to HOW TO OPEN THE AIRWAY p.34

UNCONSCIOUS CHILD (continued)

HOW TO OPEN THE AIRWAY

1 Kneel by the child's head. Place one hand on her forehead. Gently tilt her head back. As you do this, the mouth will fall open.

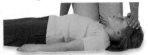

2 With your fingertips, pick out any obvious obstructions from the mouth. Do not do a finger sweep.

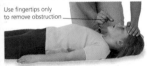

Use fingertips only to remove obstruction

3 Place the fingertips of your other hand under the point of the child's chin and gently lift the chin.

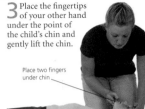

Place two fingers under chin

4 Check to see whether the child is now breathing.

▶ Go to HOW TO CHECK BREATHING below

HOW TO CHECK BREATHING

Keep the airway open and look, listen, and feel for breathing – look for chest movement, listen for sounds of breathing, and feel for breath on your cheek. Do this for no more than 10 seconds.

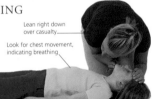

Lean right down over casualty

Look for chest movement, indicating breathing

IF THE CHILD IS BREATHING

1 Check for any life-threatening injuries such as severe bleeding. Treat as necessary.

2 Place the child in the recovery position. Regularly monitor her vital signs – level of response, pulse, and breathing (pp.8–9).

▶ Go to HOW TO PLACE IN THE RECOVERY POSITION pp.38–39

IF THE CHILD IS NOT BREATHING

1 Ask a helper to DIAL 999 FOR AN AMBULANCE.

2 Give two effective rescue breaths (right) and then check the child for signs of circulation.

▶ Go to HOW TO GIVE RESCUE BREATHS opposite

HOW TO GIVE RESCUE BREATHS

1 Ensure that the airway is still open by keeping one hand on the child's forehead and two fingers of the other hand under her chin.

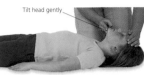

Tilt head gently

2 Pinch the soft part of the child's nose with the finger and thumb of the hand that was on the forehead. Make sure that her nostrils are closed to prevent air from escaping. Open her mouth.

Keep chin lifted

3 Take a deep breath to fill your lungs with air. Place your lips around the child's mouth, making sure that you form an airtight seal.

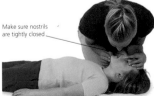

Make sure nostrils are tightly closed

4 Blow steadily into the child's mouth until the chest rises.

5 Maintaining head tilt and chin lift, take your mouth off the child's mouth and see if her chest falls. If the chest rises visibly as you blow and falls fully when you lift your mouth, you have given an effective breath. Give two effective breaths, then check for signs of circulation.

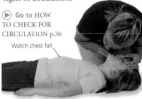

▶ Go to HOW TO CHECK FOR CIRCULATION p.36

Watch chest fall

IF YOU CANNOT ACHIEVE EFFECTIVE BREATHS

• Recheck the head tilt and chin lift.
• Recheck the child's mouth. Remove any obvious obstructions, but do not do a finger sweep of the mouth.
• Make no more than five attempts to achieve two effective breaths.
If you still cannot achieve two effective rescue breaths, check the child for signs of circulation.

▶ Go to HOW TO CHECK FOR CIRCULATION p.36

❶ WARNING

If you know that the child has choked, and you cannot achieve effective breaths, you must immediately begin giving chest compressions to try to relieve the obstruction quickly (see HOW TO GIVE CPR, pp.36–37).

35

UNCONSCIOUS CHILD (continued)

HOW TO CHECK FOR CIRCULATION

Still kneeling beside the child's head, look, listen, and feel for signs of circulation, such as breathing, coughing, or movement. Check for these signs of circulation for no more than 10 seconds.

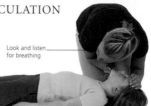

Look and listen for breathing

IF THERE ARE NO SIGNS OF CIRCULATION

Begin chest compressions and rescue breaths (cardiopulmonary resuscitation – CPR) immediately. Continue this for 1 minute then
DIAL 999 FOR AN AMBULANCE

▶ Go to HOW TO GIVE CPR below

IF YOU ARE SURE YOU HAVE DETECTED SIGNS OF CIRCULATION

1 Continue rescue breathing for 1 minute. Then **DIAL 999 FOR AN AMBULANCE.** After every 20 breaths (about 1 minute), check for signs of circulation. If the child starts to breathe but remains unconscious, place her in the recovery position (pp.38–39).

2 Monitor and record vital signs – level of response, pulse, and breathing (pp.8–9). Be prepared to turn the child on to her back again to restart rescue breathing (p.35).

HOW TO GIVE CPR

1 Kneel beside the child. With the fingertips of your lower hand, locate one of her lowermost ribs on the side nearest to you. Slide your fingertips along the rib to the point where the lowermost ribs meet at the breastbone. Place your middle finger at this point and your index finger beside it on the lower breastbone.

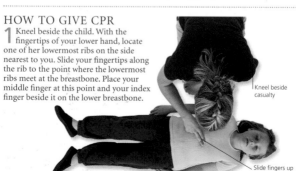

Kneel beside casualty

Slide fingers up from lowermost rib

2 Place the heel of your other hand on the breastbone and slide it down until it reaches your index finger. This is the point at which you will apply pressure.

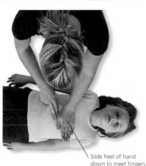

Slide heel of hand down to meet fingers

3 Use the heel of one hand only to apply pressure – keep your fingers raised so that you do not apply pressure to the child's ribs.

Keep fingers clear of chest

4 Leaning well over the child, with your arms straight, press down vertically on the breastbone and depress the chest by one-third of its depth. Release the pressure without removing your hand.

5 Compress the chest five times, at a rate of 100 compressions per minute. Compression and release should take the same amount of time.

6 Tilt the head, lift the chin, and give one rescue breath (p.35).

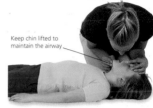

Keep chin lifted to maintain the airway

7 Continue this cycle of alternating five chest compressions with one rescue breath. Continue CPR until emergency help arrives and takes over; the child makes a movement or takes a spontaneous breath; or you become so exhausted that you cannot continue.

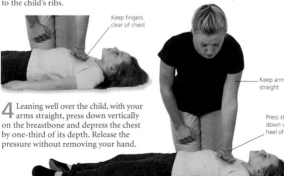

Keep arm straight

Press straight down with heel of hand

UNCONSCIOUS CHILD (continued)

HOW TO PLACE IN RECOVERY POSITION

1 Kneel beside the child. Remove any spectacles and very bulky objects from the pockets, but do not search for small items.

2 Make sure that both of the child's legs are straight. Place the arm that is nearest to you at right angles to the child's body, with the elbow bent and the palm facing upwards.

> **⚠ WARNING**
>
> If you suspect a spinal injury, and you cannot maintain the airway with the child in the position in which she was found or by using the jaw thrust method (p.81), place her in the recovery position using the guidelines opposite.

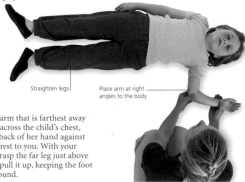

Straighten legs

Place arm at right angles to the body

3 Bring the arm that is farthest away from you across the child's chest, and hold the back of her hand against the cheek nearest to you. With your other hand, grasp the far leg just above the knee and pull it up, keeping the foot flat on the ground.

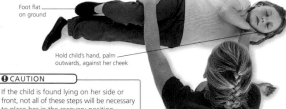

Foot flat on ground

Hold child's hand, palm outwards, against her cheek

> **⚠ CAUTION**
>
> If the child is found lying on her side or front, not all of these steps will be necessary to place her in the recovery position.

4 Keeping the child's hand pressed against her cheek, pull on the far leg and roll the child towards you and on to her side.

Tilt chin so that fluid can drain from mouth

Pull bent leg towards you

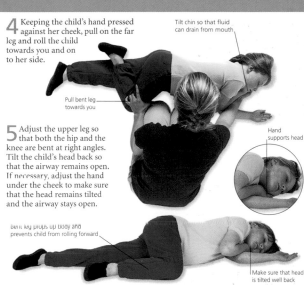

Hand supports head

5 Adjust the upper leg so that both the hip and the knee are bent at right angles. Tilt the child's head back so that the airway remains open. If necessary, adjust the hand under the cheek to make sure that the head remains tilted and the airway stays open.

Bent leg props up body and prevents child from rolling forward

Make sure that head is tilted well back

6 If it has not already been done, DIAL 999 FOR AN AMBULANCE Monitor and record vital signs – level of response, pulse, and breathing (pp.8–9) – until help arrives.

7 If the child has to be left in the recovery position for longer than 30 minutes, you should roll her on to her back, then turn her on to the opposite side – unless other injuries prevent you from doing this.

SPECIAL CASE

SPINAL INJURY

If you suspect a spinal injury, and need to place the child in the recovery position to maintain an open airway, keep the spine straight using the following guidelines:

• If you are alone, use the technique shown on this page.

• If there are two of you, one person should steady the head while the other turns the child.

• With three people, one person should steady the head while one person turns the child. The third person should keep the child's back straight during the manoeuvre.

• If there are four or more people in total, use the log-roll technique (p.81).

INFANT RESUSCITATION CHART

In infants under 1 year, a problem with breathing is the most probable reason for the heart to stop. As soon as you have established that the infant is not breathing, ask a helper to call an ambulance while you treat the infant.

CHECK INFANT'S RESPONSE
- Gently tap or flick the sole of the infant's foot. Never shake an infant.
- Is there a response?

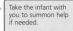

YES → Take the infant with you to summon help if needed.

NO

OPEN THE AIRWAY; CHECK FOR BREATHING
- Place one hand on the infant's forehead and very gently tilt the head back. Remove any obvious obstruction. Lift the chin. Check for breathing (p.42).
- Is the infant breathing?

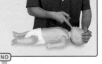

YES → Check for life-threatening injuries. Hold the infant in the recovery position (p.44) and summon help.

NO

Send a helper to **DIAL 999 FOR AN AMBULANCE**

BREATHE FOR INFANT
- Give two effective rescue breaths (pp.42–43).

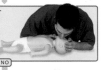

NO

> **⚠ WARNING**
>
> If you are alone, carry out rescue breathing and chest compressions for 1 minute before taking the infant with you to call an ambulance (*see* WHEN TO CALL AN AMBULANCE, p.20).

ASSESS FOR CIRCULATION
- Check for signs of circulation for no more than 10 seconds (p.43).
- Are there signs of circulation?

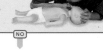

YES → Continue rescue breathing. After every 20 breaths (about 1 minute) recheck for signs of circulation. If the infant starts to breathe but remains unconscious, hold him in the recovery position (p.44).

NO

COMMENCE CPR
- Alternate five chest compressions with one rescue breath (p.44).
- Repeat as necessary.

UNCONSCIOUS INFANT (under 1 year)

The following pages give instructions for resuscitating an infant under 1 year who is apparently lifeless. (For treating an older child see pp.32–39.)

Always treat the infant from the side. You will then be in the correct position for doing all the possible stages of resuscitation.

The steps here guide you through each technique. Your first priority is to make sure that the airway is open and clear. If breathing and circulation resume, hold the infant in the recovery position (p.44). Call an ambulance immediately if an infant has known heart disease.

HOW TO CHECK FOR RESPONSE

Gently tap or flick the sole of the infant's foot and call his name to see if he responds. Never shake an infant.

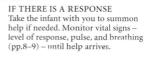

IF THERE IS A RESPONSE
Take the infant with you to summon help if needed. Monitor vital signs – level of response, pulse, and breathing (pp.8–9) – until help arrives.

IF THERE IS NO RESPONSE
Shout for help, then open the airway.

▶ Go to HOW TO OPEN THE AIRWAY below

Tap or flick sole of foot

HOW TO OPEN THE AIRWAY

1 Place a hand on the infant's forehead and very gently tilt the head back.

2 Pick out any obvious obstructions from the infant's mouth. Do not do a finger sweep.

3 Place one fingertip of the other hand under the point of the chin. Gently lift the chin. Do not push on the soft tissues under the chin as this may block the airway.

Use your fingertips to remove obstructions

Use one finger to tilt chin gently

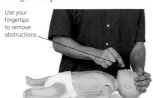

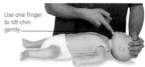

4 Check to see if the infant is now breathing.

▶ Go to HOW TO CHECK BREATHING p.42

UNCONSCIOUS INFANT (continued)

HOW TO CHECK FOR BREATHING

Keep the airway open and look, listen, and feel for breathing – look for chest movement, listen for sounds of breathing, and feel for breath on your cheek. Do this for no more than 10 seconds.

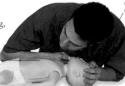

Lean right down over infant

Look for chest movement, which indicates breathing

IF THE INFANT IS BREATHING

1 Check the infant for life-threatening injuries, such as severe bleeding, and treat if necessary.

2 Hold the infant in the recovery position. Regularly monitor vital signs – level of response, pulse, and breathing (pp.8–9).

▶ Go to HOW TO HOLD IN RECOVERY POSITION p.44

IF THE INFANT IS NOT BREATHING

1 Ask a helper to DIAL 999 FOR AN AMBULANCE

2 Give two effective rescue breaths and then check for signs of circulation.

▶ Go to HOW TO GIVE RESCUE BREATHS below

HOW TO GIVE RESCUE BREATHS

1 Make sure that the airway is still open by keeping one hand on the infant's forehead and one fingertip of the other hand under the tip of his chin.

Use one finger to lift chin

2 Take a breath. Place your lips around the infant's mouth and nose to form an airtight seal. If you cannot make a seal around the mouth and nose, close the infant's mouth and make a seal around the nose only.

3 Blow steadily into the infant's lungs until the chest rises.

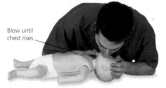

Blow until chest rises

4 Maintaining head tilt and chin lift, take your mouth off the infant's face and see if the chest falls. If the chest rises visibly as you blow and falls fully when you lift your mouth away, you have given an effective breath.

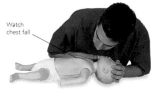

Watch chest fall

5 Give another effective rescue breath and then check for circulation.

▶ Go to HOW TO CHECK FOR CIRCULATION below

IF YOU CANNOT ACHIEVE EFFECTIVE BREATHS

- Recheck the head tilt and chin lift.
- Recheck the infant's mouth. Remove any obvious obstructions, but do not do a finger sweep of the mouth.
- Check that you have a firm seal around the mouth and nose.
- Make no more than five attempts to achieve two effective breaths. If you still cannot achieve two effective breaths, check the infant for signs of circulation.

▶ Go to HOW TO CHECK FOR CIRCULATION below

❶ WARNING

If you know that the infant has choked, and you cannot achieve effective breaths, immediately start chest compressions to try to relieve the obstruction quickly (see HOW TO GIVE CPR, p.44).

HOW TO CHECK FOR CIRCULATION

Look, listen, and feel for signs of circulation, such as breathing, coughing, or movement. Check for these signs of circulation for no more than 10 seconds.

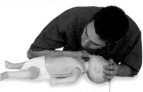

Look and listen for breathing

IF THERE ARE NO SIGNS OF CIRCULATION

Begin CPR immediately (p.44).
Continue for 1 minute, then
DIAL 999 FOR AN AMBULANCE

IF YOU ARE SURE YOU HAVE DETECTED SIGNS OF CIRCULATION

1 Continue rescue breaths for 1 minute, then
DIAL 999 FOR AN AMBULANCE
After every 20 breaths (about 1 minute), check for signs of circulation.

2 If the infant begins to breathe but remains unconscious, hold him in the recovery position.

▶ Go to HOW TO HOLD IN THE RECOVERY POSITION p.44

UNCONSCIOUS INFANT (continued)

HOW TO GIVE CPR

1 Place the infant on his back on a flat surface, at about waist height in front of you, or on the floor. Place the fingertips of your lower hand one finger's breadth below an imaginary line joining the infant's nipples. Take care not to press on the tip of the breastbone or the abdomen.

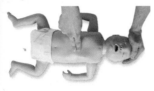

2 Press down vertically on the infant's breastbone and depress the chest by one-third of its depth. Release the pressure without losing the contact between your fingers and the breastbone.

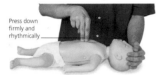

Press down firmly and rhythmically

3 Compress the chest five times, at a rate of 100 times per minute. Compression and release should take the same amount of time.

4 After five compressions, maintaining head tilt and chin lift, give one rescue breath through the mouth and nose (pp.42–43).

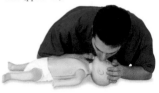

5 Continue this cycle of alternating five chest compressions with one rescue breath. Continue CPR until emergency help arrives and takes over; the infant makes a movement or takes a spontaneous breath; or you become so exhausted that you cannot continue.

HOW TO HOLD IN RECOVERY POSITION

1 Cradle the infant in your arms with his head tilted downwards. This position prevents him from choking on his tongue or inhaling vomit.

2 Monitor and record vital signs – level of response, pulse, and breathing (pp.8–9) – until help arrives.

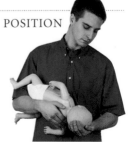

CHOKING SUMMARY CHARTS

The following pages explain how to treat a choking adult, child, or infant. The charts below summarise how to treat choking in a conscious casualty. In an adult or a child, always encourage coughing first, and start the procedures described when the casualty shows signs of weakening.

❶ WARNING

If at any stage the casualty becomes unconscious, you should open the airway, check breathing, and, if necessary, begin rescue breaths. If you cannot achieve effective breaths, begin giving chest compressions immediately to try to relieve the obstruction quickly (p.26, p.36, p.44).

PROCEDURE FOR ADULT *see* p.46

If the obstruction is still present or the casualty is getting weaker **GIVE UP TO FIVE BACK SLAPS** • Check the mouth and remove any obvious obstruction.	If the obstruction is still present **GIVE UP TO FIVE ABDOMINAL THRUSTS** • Check the mouth and remove any obvious obstruction.	If the obstruction does not clear after three cycles of back slaps and abdominal thrusts **DIAL 999 FOR AN AMBULANCE** Continue until help arrives.

PROCEDURE FOR CHILD (1–7 years) *see* p.47

If the obstruction is still present or the child is getting weaker **GIVE UP TO FIVE BACK SLAPS** • Check the mouth and remove any obvious obstruction.	If the obstruction is still present **GIVE UP TO FIVE CHEST THRUSTS** • Check the mouth and remove any obvious obstruction.	If the obstruction is still present **GIVE UP TO FIVE ABDOMINAL THRUSTS** • Check the mouth and remove any obvious obstruction.	If the obstruction does not clear after three cycles of back slaps, chest thrusts, and abdominal thrusts **DIAL 999 FOR AN AMBULANCE** Continue until help arrives.

PROCEDURE FOR INFANT (under 1 year) *see* p.48

GIVE UP TO FIVE BACK SLAPS • Check the mouth and remove any obvious obstruction.	If the obstruction is still present **GIVE UP TO FIVE CHEST THRUSTS** • Check the mouth; remove any obvious obstruction.	If the obstruction does not clear after three cycles of back slaps and chest thrusts **DIAL 999 FOR AN AMBULANCE** Continue until help arrives.

CHOKING ADULT

If blockage of the airway is partial, the casualty should be able to clear it himself; if it is complete, he will be unable to speak, breathe, or cough, and will soon lose consciousness. Be prepared to begin rescue breaths and chest compressions immediately. The throat muscles may relax slightly, leaving the airway sufficiently open for rescue breathing.

RECOGNITION

With partial obstruction:
- Coughing and distress.
- Difficulty speaking.

With complete obstruction:
- Inability to speak, breathe, or cough, and eventual loss of consciousness.

▶ See also UNCONSCIOUS ADULT pp.21–31

✚ YOUR AIMS

- To remove the obstruction.
- To arrange urgent removal to hospital if necessary.

❶ WARNING

If the casualty becomes unconscious, open the airway, check breathing, and give rescue breaths (pp.23–25). If you cannot achieve effective breaths, immediately begin giving chest compressions to try to relieve the obstruction quickly (*see* HOW TO GIVE CPR, pp.26–27).

1 If the casualty is breathing, encourage him to continue coughing. Remove any obvious obstruction from the mouth.

2 If the casualty is becoming weak, or stops breathing or coughing, carry out back slaps. Stand to the side and slightly behind him. Support his chest with one hand, and help him to lean well forwards. Give up to five sharp slaps between the shoulder blades. Stop if the obstruction clears. Check his mouth.

Use the heel of the hand to give back slaps

3 If back slaps fail to clear the obstruction, try abdominal thrusts. Stand behind the casualty and put both arms around the upper part of the abdomen. Make sure that he is still bending well forwards. Clench your fist and place it (thumb inwards) between the navel and the bottom of the breastbone. Grasp your fist with your other hand. Pull sharply inwards and upwards up to five times.

Make a fist with one hand, and position it with thumb side against the abdomen

4 Check his mouth. If the obstruction is still not cleared, repeat steps 2 and 3 up to three times, checking the mouth after each step.

5 If the obstruction still has not cleared, **DIAL 999 FOR AN AMBULANCE** Continue until help arrives or the casualty becomes unconscious.

CHOKING CHILD (1–7 years)

Young children are particularly prone to choking. A child may choke on food, or put objects into his mouth and cause a blockage of the airway.

If a child is choking, you need to act quickly. If he loses consciousness, be prepared to begin rescue breaths and chest compressions. The throat muscles may relax, leaving the airway sufficiently open for rescue breathing.

RECOGNITION

With partial obstruction:
- Coughing and distress.
- Difficulty speaking.

With complete obstruction:
- Inability to speak, breathe, or cough, and eventual loss of consciousness.

See also UNCONSCIOUS CHILD pp.33–39

+ YOUR AIMS

- To remove the obstruction.
- To arrange urgent removal to hospital if necessary.

1 If the child is breathing, encourage him to cough; this may be enough to clear the obstruction.

2 If the child shows signs of becoming weak, or stops breathing or coughing, carry out back slaps. Bend him well forwards and give up to five slaps between his shoulder blades using the heel of your hand. Check his mouth.

3 If back slaps fail to dislodge the obstruction, try chest thrusts. Stand or kneel behind the child. Place a fist (thumb inwards) against the lower half of his breastbone. Grasp the fist with your other hand. Pull sharply inwards and upwards. Give up to five chest thrusts, at a rate of one every 3 seconds. Stop if the obstruction clears. Check his mouth.

Make sure that child is bending well forwards

4 If the chest thrusts fail, try abdominal thrusts. Put your arms around the child's upper abdomen. Make sure that he is bending well forwards. Place your fist between the navel and the bottom of the breastbone, and grasp it with your other hand. Pull sharply inwards and upwards up to five times. Stop if the obstruction clears. Check his mouth.

Fist should be just above child's navel

5 If the obstruction is still not cleared, repeat steps 2–4 up to three times.

6 If the obstruction has still not cleared, DIAL 999 FOR AN AMBULANCE Continue until help arrives or the child becomes unconscious.

! WARNING

If at any stage the child becomes unconscious, open the airway, check breathing, and give rescue breaths (pp.34–35). If you cannot achieve effective breaths, immediately begin giving chest compressions to try to relieve the obstruction quickly (*see* HOW TO GIVE CPR, pp.36–37).

CHOKING INFANT (under 1 year)

An infant may readily choke on food or small objects. He will rapidly become distressed, and you need to act fast. If he becomes unconscious, be prepared to give rescue breaths and chest compressions. When he is unconscious, the throat muscles may relax, opening the airway for rescue breathing, and chest compressions may clear the obstruction.

RECOGNITION

With partial obstruction:
- Coughing and distress.
- Difficulty crying or making any other noise.

With complete obstruction:
- Inability to breathe or cough, and eventual loss of consciousness.

▶ See also UNCONSCIOUS INFANT pp.41–44

✚ YOUR AIMS

- To remove the obstruction.
- To arrange urgent removal to hospital if necessary.

❶ WARNING

If the infant becomes unconscious, open the airway, check breathing, and give rescue breaths (pp.41–43). If you cannot achieve effective breaths, immediately begin chest compressions to try to relieve the obstruction quickly (*see* HOW TO GIVE CPR, p.44).

1 If the infant is distressed, shows signs of becoming weak, or stops breathing or coughing, lay him face down along your forearm, with his head low, and support his back and head. Give up to five back slaps.

Make sure that head is below level of chest

2 Check the infant's mouth; remove any obvious obstructions with your fingertips. Do not do a finger sweep of the mouth.

3 If this fails to clear the obstruction, turn the infant on to his back and give up to five chest thrusts. Using two fingers, push inwards and upwards (towards the head) against the infant's breastbone, one finger's breadth below the nipple line.

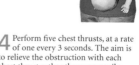

Push on breastbone with your fingertips, one finger's breadth below nipple line

4 Perform five chest thrusts, at a rate of one every 3 seconds. The aim is to relieve the obstruction with each chest thrust rather than necessarily doing all five. Check the mouth.

5 If the obstruction is not cleared, repeat steps 1–4 three times. If the obstruction still has not cleared, take the infant with you to **DIAL 999 FOR AN AMBULANCE** Continue until help arrives or the infant becomes unconscious.

3

T HE HEART and the network of
blood vessels, collectively known
as the circulatory (cardiovascular)
system, pump blood around the body,
carrying oxygen and nutrients to all
body tissues. The structures that
enable us to breathe, or take in oxygen
and expel carbon dioxide, make up
the respiratory system.

WHAT CAN GO WRONG
The circulatory system may be
disrupted in two main ways: severe
bleeding and fluid loss may cause the
volume of blood to fall, depriving the
organs of oxygen; or age or disease
may cause the system to break down.
Respiration can be impaired in various
ways. The airways may be blocked; the
lungs may be affected by inhalation of
smoke or fumes or impaired by chest
injury; or breathing may be affected
by conditions such as asthma.

CONTENTS

Shock 50

Anaphylactic shock 52

Angina pectoris..................... 53

Acute heart failure 53

Heart attack.......................... 54

Fainting................................ 55

Asthma 56

Drowning.............................. 57

Penetrating chest wound 58

✚ FIRST-AID PRIORITIES

- Assess the casualty's condition.
- Comfort and reassure the casualty.
- Maintain an open airway, check
breathing, and be prepared to resuscitate
if necessary.
- Obtain medical aid if necessary. Call an
ambulance if you suspect a serious illness
or injury.

CIRCULATORY AND RESPIRATORY PROBLEMS

SHOCK

This life-threatening condition requires immediate emergency treatment to prevent permanent organ damage and death. It can be made worse by fear and pain. Where there is a risk of shock developing, reassuring the casualty and making her comfortable may be sufficient to prevent her from deteriorating.

CAUSES OF SHOCK
The most common cause of shock is severe blood loss. If this exceeds 1.2 litres (2 pints) shock will occur. Such blood loss may result from wounds or be due to bleeding from internal organs, blood escaping into a body cavity, or bleeding from damaged blood vessels due to a fracture (p.70).

Shock can also result from loss of other body fluids due to diarrhoea, vomiting, blockage in the intestine, or severe burns. It may occur when the heart is unable to pump blood, perhaps due to severe heart disease, heart attack, or acute heart failure.

Other causes of shock include overwhelming infection, lack of certain hormones, low blood sugar

(hypoglycaemia), hypothermia, severe allergic reaction (anaphylactic shock), drug overdose, and spinal cord injury.

RECOGNITION

Initially:
• A rapid pulse.
• Pale, cold, clammy skin; sweating.
As shock develops:
• Grey–blue skin (cyanosis), especially inside the lips. A fingernail or earlobe, if pressed, will not regain its colour immediately.
• Weakness and dizziness.
• Nausea, and possibly vomiting.
• Thirst.
• Rapid, shallow breathing.
• A weak, "thready" pulse. When the pulse at the wrist disappears, about half of the blood volume will have been lost.
As the brain's oxygen supply weakens:
• Restlessness and aggressiveness.
• Yawning and gasping for air.
• Unconsciousness.
Finally, the heart will stop.

▶ See also ANAPHYLACTIC SHOCK p.52
• LIFE-SAVING PROCEDURES pp.19–48
• SEVERE BLEEDING pp.60–61
• SEVERE BURNS AND SCALDS pp.98–99

EFFECTS OF BLOOD OR FLUID LOSS	
Approximate volume lost	Effects on the body
0.5 litre (about 1 pint)	Little or no effect; this is the quantity normally taken in a blood-donor session
Up to 2 litres (3.5 pints)	Hormones such as adrenaline are released, quickening the pulse and inducing sweating • Small blood vessels in non-vital areas, such as the skin, shut down to divert blood and oxygen to the vital organs • Shock becomes evident
2 litres (3.5 pints) or more (over a third of the normal volume in the average adult)	As blood or fluid loss approaches this level, the pulse at the wrist may become undetectable • Casualty will usually lose consciousness • Breathing may cease and the heart may stop

1 Treat any possible cause of shock that you can detect, such as severe bleeding (pp.60–61) or serious burns (p.98).

2 Lay the casualty down on a blanket to insulate her from the cold ground. Constantly reassure her.

3 Raise and support her legs to improve the blood supply to the vital organs. Take care if you suspect a fracture.

Keeping head low may prevent casualty losing consciousness

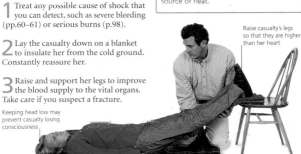

Raise casualty's legs so that they are higher than their heart

4 Loosen tight clothing at the neck, chest, and waist to reduce constriction in these areas.

5 Keep the casualty warm by covering her body and legs with coats or blankets. **DIAL 999 FOR AN AMBULANCE**

6 Monitor and record vital signs – level of response, pulse, and breathing (pp.8–9). If the casualty becomes unconscious, open the airway and check breathing; be prepared to give rescue breaths and chest compressions if necessary (see LIFE-SAVING PROCEDURES, pp.19–48).

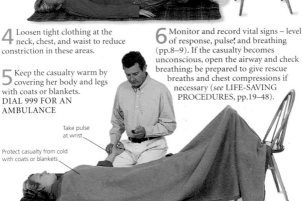

Take pulse at wrist

Protect casualty from cold with coats or blankets

ANAPHYLACTIC SHOCK

A severe and potentially fatal allergic reaction, anaphylactic shock may develop within seconds or minutes of contact with a trigger, including:

● Skin or airborne contact with particular materials.

● The injection of a specific drug.

● The sting of a certain insect.

● Ingestion of a food such as peanuts. Chemicals are released into the blood that widen (dilate) blood vessels and constrict (narrow) air passages. Blood pressure falls, breathing is impaired, the tongue and throat may swell, and the vital organs are starved of oxygen.

A casualty needs emergency treatment with an injection of epinephrine (adrenaline). Priorities are to ease breathing and minimise shock until specialised help arrives.

✚ YOUR AIM

● To arrange urgent removal to hospital.

❶ WARNING

If the casualty becomes unconscious, open the airway and check breathing; be prepared to give rescue breaths and chest compressions if necessary (see LIFE-SAVING PROCEDURES, pp.19–48). If the casualty is breathing, place her in the recovery position (pp.30–31).

1 DIAL 999 FOR AN AMBULANCE Give any information you have on the cause of the casualty's condition.

2 Check whether the casualty has the necessary medication – a syringe or an auto-injector of epinephrine (adrenaline) for self-administration. Help her to use it. If the casualty is unable to administer the medication, and you have been trained to use an auto-injector, give it to her yourself.

3 If the casualty is conscious, help her to sit up in the position that most relieves any breathing difficulty.

4 Treat the casualty for shock (pp.50–51) if necessary.

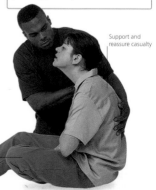

Support and reassure casualty

Sitting position should help to ease casualty's breathing

ANGINA PECTORIS

Meaning "a constriction of the chest", angina pectoris occurs when coronary arteries, which supply the heart muscle with blood, become narrowed and cannot carry sufficient blood to meet increased demands during exertion or excitement. An attack forces the casualty to rest; the pain should ease soon afterwards.

- Vice-like central chest pain, often spreading to the jaw and down one or both arms.
- Pain easing with rest.
- Shortness of breath.
- Weakness, often sudden and extreme.
- Feeling of anxiety.

YOUR AIMS

- To ease strain on the heart by ensuring that the casualty rests.
- To obtain medical help if necessary.
- To help the casualty with any medication.

WARNING

If the pain persists, or returns, suspect a heart attack (p.54)

DIAL 999 FOR AN AMBULANCE

Treat by giving the casualty a full-dose (300 mg) aspirin tablet to chew. Constantly monitor and record vital signs – level of response, pulse, and breathing (pp.8–9).

If the casualty becomes unconscious, open the airway and check breathing; be prepared to give rescue breaths and chest compressions if necessary (see LIFE-SAVING PROCEDURES, pp.19–48).

1 Help the casualty to sit down. Make sure she is comfortable and reassure her. This should help her breathing.

2 If the casualty has medication for angina, such as tablets or a pump-action or aerosol spray, let her administer it herself. If necessary, help her to take it

Supervise and support casualty as she takes medication

3 Encourage the casualty to rest, and keep any bystanders away. The attack should ease within a few minutes.

ACUTE HEART FAILURE

In heart failure, the heart muscle is over-strained or damaged and cannot pump sufficient blood to the body. Fluid may build up in the lungs, making breathing difficult. A possible cause is a clot in a coronary artery (coronary thrombosis). Heart failure occurs suddenly, often at night.

- Severe breathlessness.
- Often, but not always, signs and symptoms of heart attack (p.54).

▶ Treat as for HEART ATTACK p.54

HEART ATTACK

A heart attack is most commonly caused by a sudden obstruction of the blood supply to part of the heart muscle. The main risk is that the heart will stop beating.

The effects of a heart attack depend largely on how much of the heart muscle is affected; many casualties recover completely. Drugs such as aspirin, and medications that dissolve the clot, are used to limit the extent of damage to the heart muscle.

> See also LIFE-SAVING PROCEDURES pp.19–48

pp.19–48

RECOGNITION

- Persistent, vice-like central chest pain, often spreading to the jaw and down one or both arms. Unlike angina pectoris (p.53), the pain does not ease if the casualty rests.
- Breathlessness, and discomfort occurring high in the abdomen, which may feel similar to severe indigestion.
- Collapse, often without any warning.
- Sudden faintness or dizziness.
- A sense of impending doom.
- "Ashen" skin, and blueness at the lips.
- A rapid, weak, or irregular pulse.
- Profuse sweating.
- Extreme gasping for air ("air hunger").

+ YOUR AIMS

- To encourage the casualty to rest.
- To arrange urgent removal of the casualty to hospital.

! WARNING

If the casualty becomes unconscious, open the airway and check breathing; be prepared to give rescue breaths and chest compressions if needed (see LIFE-SAVING PROCEDURES, pp.19–48).

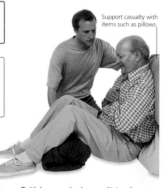

Support casualty with items such as pillows

1 Make the casualty as comfortable as possible to ease the strain on his heart. A half-sitting position, with head and shoulders well supported and knees bent, is often best.

2 DIAL 999 FOR AN AMBULANCE State that you suspect a heart attack. If the casualty asks you to do so, call his own doctor as well.

3 If the casualty is fully conscious, give him a full-dose (300 mg) aspirin tablet and advise him to chew it slowly.

4 If the casualty has medicine for angina, such as tablets or a pump-action or aerosol spray, help him to take it. Encourage the casualty to rest.

5 Constantly monitor and record vital signs – level of response, pulse, and breathing (pp.8–9) – until help arrives.

FAINTING

A faint is a brief loss of consciousness caused by a temporary reduction of the blood flow to the brain. Fainting may be a reaction to pain, exhaustion, lack of food, or emotional stress. It is also common after long periods of inactivity, such as standing or sitting still, especially in a warm atmosphere – blood pools in the legs, reducing the amount reaching the brain.

When a person faints, the pulse rate becomes very slow. However, the rate

soon picks up and returns to normal. A casualty who has fainted usually makes a rapid and complete recovery.

> See also LIFE-SAVING PROCEDURES pp.19–48

RECOGNITION
- A brief loss of consciousness that causes the casualty to fall to the floor.
- A slow pulse.
- Pale, cold skin and sweating.

+ YOUR AIMS
- To improve blood flow to the brain.
- To reassure the casualty as she recovers and make her comfortable.

1 When a casualty feels faint, advise her to lie down. Kneel down, raise her legs, and support her ankles on your shoulders; this helps to improve the blood flow to the brain.

Support ankles on your shoulders

Raise legs to improve blood flow to brain

Watch face for signs of recovery

2 Make sure that the casualty has plenty of fresh air; ask someone to open a window. In addition, ask any bystanders to stand clear.

3 As she recovers, reassure her and help her to sit up gradually. If she starts to feel faint again, advise her to lie down again, and raise and support her legs until she recovers fully.

! WARNING
If the casualty does not regain consciousness quickly, open the airway and check breathing; be prepared to give rescue breaths and chest compressions if necessary (see LIFE-SAVING PROCEDURES, pp.19–48).

DIAL 999 FOR AN AMBULANCE

ASTHMA

In an asthma attack, the muscles of the air passages in the lungs go into spasm and the linings of the airways swell. The airways become narrowed, making breathing difficult.

Sufferers usually treat their own attacks, using a "reliever" inhaler (most have blue caps). A diffuser or "spacer" can be fitted to help administer the medication. Preventer inhalers (with brown or white caps) are used with sufferers to help prevent attacks. Preventer inhalers are not an effective treatment for asthma attacks.

RECOGNITION

- Difficulty in breathing, with a very prolonged breathing-out phase.

There may also be:
- Wheezing as the casualty breathes out.
- Difficulty speaking and whispering.
- Features of hypoxia, such as a grey–blue tinge to the lips, earlobes, and nailbeds (cyanosis).
- Distress and anxiety.
- Cough.
- In a severe attack, exhaustion. Rarely, the casualty loses consciousness and stops breathing.

+ YOUR AIMS

- To ease breathing.
- To obtain medical help if necessary.

1 Keep calm and reassure the casualty. Get her to take a puff of her reliever inhaler. It should relieve the asthma attack within a few minutes. Ask her to breathe slowly and deeply.

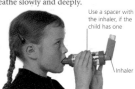

Use a spacer with the inhaler, if the child has one

Inhaler

2 Let her adopt the position that she finds most comfortable – often sitting down. Do not make the casualty lie down.

3 A mild asthma attack should ease within 3 minutes. If it does not, ask the casualty to take another dose from the same inhaler.

! CAUTION

If this is the first attack, or if the attack is severe and any one of the following occurs:
- the inhaler has no effect after 5 minutes,
- the casualty is getting worse,
- breathlessness makes talking difficult,
- she is becoming exhausted,

DIAL 999 FOR AN AMBULANCE

Help her to use her inhaler every 5–10 minutes. Monitor and record her breathing and pulse every 10 minutes (pp.8–9).

! WARNING

If the casualty loses consciousness, open the airway and check breathing; be prepared to give rescue breaths and chest compressions if necessary (see LIFE-SAVING PROCEDURES, pp.19–48).

DIAL 999 FOR AN AMBULANCE

If the casualty is breathing, place her in the recovery position (pp.30–31). Monitor her vital signs – level of response, pulse, and breathing (pp.8–9) – until help arrives.

DROWNING

Death by drowning occurs when air cannot get into the lungs, usually because of a small amount of water. This may also cause throat spasms.

Water may gush from the mouth of a rescued casualty. It is from the stomach and should be left to drain of its own accord. Do not attempt to force it from the stomach because the casualty may vomit and then inhale it. A casualty should always receive medical attention even if he seems to recover at the time. Water in the lungs causes them to become irritated, and the air passages may begin to swell several hours later – a condition known as secondary drowning.

Casualties may also need treatment for hypothermia (pp.108–110).

▶ See also HYPOTHERMIA pp.108–110
● LIFE-SAVING PROCEDURES pp.19–48

+ YOUR AIMS

- To restore adequate breathing.
- To keep the casualty warm
- To arrange urgent removal to hospital.

1 If you are rescuing the casualty from the water to safety, keep her head lower than the rest of the body to reduce the risk of her inhaling water.

2 Lay the casualty down on her back on a rug or coat. Open the airway and check breathing; be prepared to give rescue breaths and chest compressions if necessary (see LIFE-SAVING PROCEDURES, pp.19–48). If the casualty is breathing, place her in the recovery position (pp.30–31).

Listen and feel for breathing

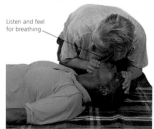

3 Treat the casualty for hypothermia; remove wet clothing if possible and cover her with dry blankets. If the casualty regains full consciousness, give her a warm drink.

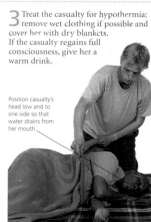

Position casualty's head low and to one side so that water drains from her mouth

4 DIAL 999 FOR AN AMBULANCE even if she appears to recover fully.

❶ WARNING

Water in the lungs and the effects of cold can increase resistance to rescue breaths and chest compressions: you may have to do both at a slower rate than normal.

PENETRATING CHEST WOUND

The heart and lungs, and the major blood vessels around them, lie within the chest (thorax), protected by the breastbone and the ribcage, which extends downwards to protect organs such as the liver and spleen in the upper abdomen. Penetrating wounds can cause severe internal damage. The lungs are particularly susceptible and damage to them causes breathing difficulties; it may also impair the operation of the heart, causing shock.

▶ See also LIFE-SAVING PROCEDURES pp.19–48 ● SHOCK pp.50–51

RECOGNITION

- Difficult and painful breathing, possibly rapid, shallow, and uneven.
- Casualty feels an acute sense of alarm.
- Features of hypoxia, including grey–blue skin coloration (cyanosis).

There may also be:
- Coughed-up frothy, red blood.
- A crackling feeling of the skin around the site of the wound, caused by air collecting in the tissues.
- Blood bubbling out of the wound.
- Sound of air being sucked into the chest as the casualty breathes in.
- Veins in the neck becoming prominent.

✚ YOUR AIMS

- To seal the wound and maintain breathing.
- To minimise shock.
- To arrange urgent removal to hospital.

❶ WARNING

If the casualty becomes unconscious, open the airway and check breathing; be prepared to give rescue breaths and chest compressions, if necessary (see LIFE-SAVING PROCEDURES, pp.19–48). If breathing, place him in the recovery position (pp.30–31) on his injured side to help the healthy lung to work effectively.

1 Put on disposable gloves if available. Lean the casualty towards the injured side and cover the wound with his palm.

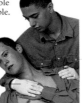

Completely cover the wound to stop air from being drawn into the chest cavity

2 Place a sterile dressing or non-fluffy clean pad over the wound and surrounding area. Cover with a plastic bag, foil, or kitchen film. Secure firmly with adhesive tape on three edges, or with bandages around the chest, so that the dressing is taut.

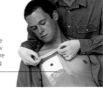

Leave fourth side untaped to allow air under pressure during breathing out to escape

3 DIAL 999 FOR AN AMBULANCE While waiting for help, continue to support the casualty in the same position as long as he remains conscious.

4 Monitor and record vital signs – level of response, pulse, and breathing (pp.8–9) – until medical help arrives.

4

B REAKS IN THE SKIN or the body
surfaces are known as wounds.
Open wounds allow blood and other
fluids to be lost from the body and
enable germs to enter. In a closed
wound, bleeding is confined within
the body tissues and is most easily
recognised by bruising. Wounds can
be daunting, particularly if there is a
lot of bleeding, but prompt action will
reduce blood loss and minimise shock.

UNDERSTANDING TREATMENT
The way in which injury is inflicted
and the force exerted determine the
effect of the wound on the body and
how to treat it. Treatments for all
types of wound are covered in this
chapter. Always follow good hygiene
procedures to guard against cross-
infection: wash your hands and wear
disposable gloves if available.

✚ FIRST-AID PRIORITIES

- Assess the casualty's condition.
- Comfort and reassure the casualty.
- Take care with hygiene.
- Control blood loss by applying
  pressure and elevating the injured part.
- Minimise shock.
- Obtain medical help, if necessary.
  Call an ambulance if you suspect a
  serious illness or injury.

CONTENTS

Severe bleeding 60

Cuts and grazes....................62

Foreign object in a cut 63

Scalp and head wounds..........64

Eye wound............................65

Bleeding from the ear 65

Nosebleed.............................66

Abdominal wound 67

Wound to the palm 68

Wound at a joint crease..........68

WOUNDS AND BLEEDING

SEVERE BLEEDING

When bleeding is severe, it can be dramatic and distressing. Shock is likely to develop, and the casualty may lose consciousness. If bleeding is not controlled, the casualty's heart could stop. Bleeding at the face or neck may impede the air flow to the lungs.

When treating severe bleeding, always check first whether there is an object embedded in the wound; take care not to press on the object.

▶ See also LIFE-SAVING PROCEDURES pp.19–48 ● SHOCK pp.50–51

IF NO OBJECT IS EMBEDDED IN WOUND

+ YOUR AIMS

- To control bleeding.
- To prevent/minimise the effects of shock.
- To minimise infection.
- To arrange urgent removal to hospital.

1 Put on disposable gloves if available. Remove or cut clothing as necessary to expose the wound.

2 Apply direct pressure over the wound with your fingers or palm, preferably over a sterile dressing or non-fluffy, clean pad (but do not waste any time by looking for a dressing). You can ask the casualty to apply direct pressure herself.

3 Raise and support the injured limb above the level of the casualty's heart to reduce blood loss. Handle the limb very gently if you suspect that there is a fracture.

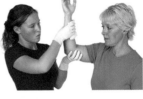

4 Help the casualty to lie down on a blanket, if available, to protect her from the cold. If you suspect that shock may develop, raise and support her legs so that they are above the level of her heart.

Keep injured limb raised

Maintain pressure on dressing

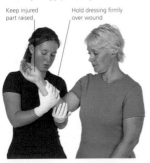

Keep injured part raised

Hold dressing firmly over wound

5 Secure the dressing with a bandage that is tight enough to maintain pressure, but not so tight that it impairs the circulation (p.14). If further bleeding occurs, apply a second dressing on top of the first.

If using a pad, cover it completely with bandage

6 If blood seeps through the second dressing, remove both dressings and apply a fresh one, applying pressure accurately to the point of bleeding.

7 Support the injured part and keep it raised with a sling and/or bandaging.

8 DIAL 999 FOR AN AMBULANCE Regularly monitor and record vital signs – level of response, pulse, and breathing (pp.8–9). Watch for signs of shock (pp.50–51), and check the dressings for seepage. Always check the circulation beyond the bandage (p.14).

❶ CAUTION

Do not give the casualty anything to eat, drink, or smoke.

IF AN OBJECT IS EMBEDDED IN WOUND

✚ YOUR AIMS

- To control bleeding without pressing the object into the wound.
- To prevent/minimise the effects of shock.
- To minimise infection.
- To arrange urgent removal to hospital.

1 Put on disposable gloves if available. Press firmly on either side of the wound to push the edges of the wound together.

2 If the injury is to a casualty's limb, raise and support the limb above the level of her heart to reduce the blood loss.

3 If possible, help the casualty to lie down on a blanket to protect her from the cold. If you suspect that shock may develop, raise and support her legs so that they are above the level of her heart.

4 Build up padding on either side of the object. Carefully bandage over the object without pressing on it.

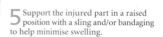

Take care not to press on object

5 Support the injured part in a raised position with a sling and/or bandaging to help minimise swelling.

6 DIAL 999 FOR AN AMBULANCE Monitor and record vital signs – level of response, pulse, and breathing (pp.8–9). Watch for signs of shock (pp.50–51), and check the dressing for seepage. Check the circulation beyond the bandage (p.14).

CUTS AND GRAZES

Bleeding from small cuts and grazes is controlled by pressure and elevation. An adhesive dressing is normally all that is necessary, and the wound will heal in a few days. Medical aid need only be sought if:

● The bleeding does not stop.
● There is a foreign object embedded in the cut (opposite).
● The wound is at particular risk of infection (such as a human or animal bite, or a puncture by a dirty object).
● An old wound shows signs of becoming infected.

TETANUS

This is a dangerous infection caused by the bacterium *Clostridium tetani*. If tetanus bacteria enter a wound, they may multiply and release a poisonous substance (toxin) that spreads through the nervous system, causing muscle spasms and paralysis.

The disorder can be prevented by immunisation, and people are normally given a course of tetanus immunisation during childhood. However, immunisation may need to be repeated in adulthood.

✚ YOUR AIM

● To minimise the risk of infection.

1 Wash your hands thoroughly, and put on disposable gloves if available.

2 If the wound is dirty, clean it by rinsing lightly under running water, or use an alcohol-free wipe. Then pat the wound dry using a gauze swab and cover with sterile gauze.

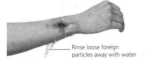

Rinse loose foreign particles away with water

❶ CAUTION

Always ask about tetanus immunisation.
Seek medical advice if:
● The casualty has never been immunised.
● The casualty is uncertain about the timing and number of injections given.
● It is more than 10 years since the casualty's last injection.

3 Elevate the injured part above the level of the heart, if possible. Avoid touching the wound directly. Support the affected limb with one hand.

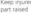

Keep injured part raised

4 Clean the surrounding area with soap and water; use clean swabs for each stroke. Pat dry. Remove the wound covering and apply an adhesive dressing. If there is a special risk of infection, advise the casualty to see her doctor.

Wipe away from wound, using a clean gauze swab for each stroke

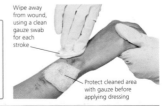

Protect cleaned area with gauze before applying dressing

FOREIGN OBJECT IN A CUT

Always remove foreign objects, such as small pieces of glass or grit, from wounds before giving treatment. If such items remain in a wound, they may cause infection or delayed healing in the short term and discoloration in the long term. Remove superficial pieces of glass or grit with tweezers. Alternatively, carefully pick the pieces off the wound or rinse them off with cold water. Do not remove objects that are firmly embedded in the wound because you may damage tissue and aggravate bleeding. Instead, apply dressings or bandages around them.

▶ See also EMBEDDED FISH-HOOK p.113
● SPLINTER p.112

+ YOUR AIMS

- To control bleeding without pressing the object into the wound.
- To minimise the risk of infection.
- To arrange transport to hospital if needed.

1 Put on disposable gloves if available. Control any bleeding by applying pressure on either side of the object and raising the injured part above heart level.

2 Cover the wound with gauze to minimise the risk of infection.

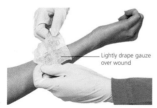

Lightly drape gauze over wound

⊘ CAUTION

Always ask about tetanus immunisation.
Seek medical advice if:
- The casualty has never been immunised.
- The casualty is uncertain about the timing and number of injections given.
- It is more than 10 years since the casualty's last injection.

3 Build up padding around the object until you are able to bandage over it without pressing down. Carefully hold the padding in place until you have completed the bandaging.

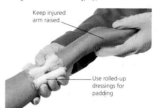

Keep injured arm raised

Use rolled-up dressings for padding

4 Arrange to take or send the casualty to hospital if necessary.

SPECIAL CASE

LARGE OBJECTS
If the object is particularly large, and you cannot pad high enough to bandage over it without pressing on it, bandage around the object.

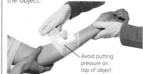

Avoid putting pressure on top of object

SCALP AND HEAD WOUNDS

The scalp has many small blood vessels close to the skin surface, so any cut can lead to profuse bleeding. This bleeding will often make a scalp wound appear worse than it is. However, in some cases, a scalp wound may form part of a more serious underlying injury, such as a skull fracture, or may be associated with a head or neck injury. For these reasons, you should examine a casualty with a scalp wound very carefully, particularly if signs of a serious head injury may be masked by alcohol or drug intoxication. If you are in any doubt, follow the treatment for skull fracture (p.90). Also bear in mind the possibility of a neck (spinal) injury.

▶ See also SHOCK pp.50–51 ● SKULL FRACTURE p.90 ● SPINAL INJURY pp.79–81

✚ YOUR AIMS

● To control blood loss.
● To arrange transport to hospital.

❶ WARNING

If the casualty becomes unconscious, open the airway and check breathing; be prepared to give rescue breaths and chest compressions if necessary (see LIFE-SAVING PROCEDURES, pp.19–48).

1 Put on disposable gloves if available. If there are any displaced flaps of skin at the injury site, carefully replace them over the wound. Reassure the casualty.

2 Cover the injury with a sterile wound dressing or a clean, non-fluffy pad. Apply firm, direct pressure on the pad. This measure will help control bleeding and reduce blood loss, minimising the risk of shock developing.

3 Secure the dressing with a roller bandage. (For minor bleeding, you can keep the pad in place with a triangular bandage.)

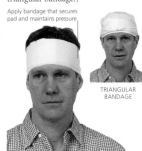

Apply bandage that secures pad and maintains pressure

TRIANGULAR BANDAGE

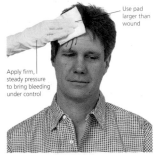

Use pad larger than wound

Apply firm, steady pressure to bring bleeding under control

4 Help the casualty lie down, with his head and shoulders slightly raised. Take or send the casualty to hospital in the final treatment position. Regularly monitor and record the level of response, pulse, and breathing (pp.8–9).

EYE WOUND

The eye can be bruised or cut by direct blows or by sharp, chipped fragments of metal, grit, and glass.

All eye injuries are potentially serious because of the risk to the casualty's vision. Even superficial grazes to the surface (cornea) of the eye can lead to scarring or infection. Do not touch or attempt to remove a foreign object that is embedded in the eye (p.114).

RECOGNITION

- Intense pain and spasm of the eyelids.
- Visible wound and/or bloodshot eye.
- Partial or total loss of vision.
- Leakage of blood or clear fluid from a wound.

See also FOREIGN OBJECT IN THE EYE p.114

YOUR AIMS

- To prevent further damage.
- To arrange transport to hospital.

1 Help the casualty to lie on her back, and hold her head to keep it as still as possible. Tell her to keep both eyes still; movement of the "good" eye will cause movement of the injured one, which may damage it further.

2 Ask the casualty to hold a sterile wound dressing or clean, non-fluffy pad over the eye. If it will take time to obtain medical help, secure the pad with a bandage. Take or send the casualty to hospital in the treatment position.

Use a large, soft pad that covers eye

BLEEDING FROM THE EAR

This usually occurs when an eardrum is burst (perforated), perhaps caused by a foreign object pushed in the ear, a blow to the side of the head, or an explosion. Symptoms include sharp pain, earache, deafness, and possible dizziness. Watery blood is serious: it indicates that the skull is fractured and fluid is leaking from around the brain.

See also FOREIGN OBJECT IN THE EAR p.115 • SKULL FRACTURE p.90

YOUR AIM

- To arrange transport to hospital.

CAUTION

Do not tilt the casualty's head if you suspect a skull fracture.

1 Help the casualty into a half-sitting position, with his head tilted to the injured side so that blood drains away.

2 Put on gloves if available. Hold a sterile wound dressing or a clean, non-fluffy pad lightly in place on the ear. Send or take the casualty to hospital in the treatment position.

NOSEBLEED

Bleeding from the nose often occurs when blood vessels inside the nostrils rupture, perhaps as a result of sneezing or blowing the nose. Nosebleeds may also occur as a result of high blood pressure. A nosebleed can be dangerous if the casualty loses a lot of blood.

If bleeding follows a head injury and the blood is thin and watery, this is serious: fluid leaking from around the brain indicates a fractured skull.

▶ See also FOREIGN OBJECT IN THE NOSE p.115

YOUR AIMS

• To control blood loss.
• To maintain an open airway.

1 Ask the casualty to sit down. Advise her to tilt her head forwards to allow the blood to drain from the nostrils.

2 Ask the casualty to breathe through her mouth (this will also have a calming effect) and to pinch the soft part of the nose. Reassure and help her if necessary.

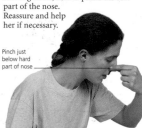

Pinch just below hard part of nose

SPECIAL CASE

CHILDREN
A young child may well be worried by a nosebleed. Try to reassure her and give her a bowl that she can spit or dribble into.

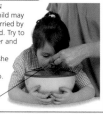

Pinch child's nose

3 Tell the casualty to keep pinching her nose. Advise her not to speak, swallow, cough, spit, or sniff because she may disturb blood clots that have formed in the nose. Give her a clean cloth or tissue to mop up any dribbling.

4 After about 10 minutes, tell the casualty to release the pressure. If the bleeding has not stopped, tell her to reapply the pressure for two further periods of 10 minutes.

5 Once the bleeding has stopped, and with the casualty still leaning forwards, clean around her nose with lukewarm water.

6 Advise the casualty to rest quietly for a few hours. Tell her to avoid exertion and, in particular, not to blow her nose, because these actions will disturb any clots.

❗ CAUTION

• Do not let the head tip back; blood may run down the throat and induce vomiting.
• If bleeding stops and then restarts, tell the casualty to reapply pressure.
• If the nosebleed is severe, or if it lasts longer than 30 minutes in total, take or send the casualty to hospital in the treatment position.

ABDOMINAL WOUND

A knife, gunshot, or crush injury to the abdomen can puncture, lacerate or rupture organs and major blood vessels deep inside the body. The severity of a wound may be evident from symptoms such as external bleeding and protruding abdominal contents. More often, there is hidden internal injury and bleeding, which may be fatal if there is any delay in emergency treatment. There is also a high risk of shock and infection.

See also SHOCK pp.50–51

+ YOUR AIMS

- To minimise shock.
- To minimise the risk of infection.
- To arrange urgent removal to hospital.

1 Put on disposable gloves if available. Help the casualty to lie down on a firm surface, preferably on a blanket. Loosen any tight clothing, such as a belt or a shirt.

Undo belt

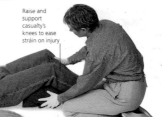

Raise and support casualty's knees to ease strain on injury

3 DIAL 999 FOR AN AMBULANCE Treat the casualty for shock (pp.50–51). Regularly monitor and record vital signs – level of response, pulse, and breathing (pp.8–9).

2 Put a dressing over the wound, and secure it in place with a bandage or adhesive tape. If blood seeps through the dressing, apply another dressing or pad on top of the first one.

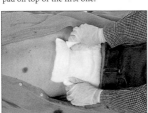

⚠ WARNING

- If a casualty with an open wound coughs or vomits, press on the dressing to prevent the contents of the abdomen from pushing through the wound and being exposed.

- Do not touch any protruding intestine. Cover the area with a clean plastic bag or kitchen film. Alternatively, apply a sterile wound dressing.

- If the casualty becomes unconscious, open the airway and check breathing; be ready to give rescue breaths and chest compressions if needed (see LIFE-SAVING PROCEDURES, pp.19–48). If he is breathing, put him in the recovery position (pp.30–31), taking care to support the abdomen.

WOUND TO THE PALM

Because the palm has several large blood vessels, a wound here may cause profuse bleeding. There is also a risk that a deep wound to the palm may sever tendons and nerves in the hand and result in loss of feeling or movement in the fingers.

▶ See also FOREIGN OBJECT IN A CUT p.63
● SHOCK pp.50–51

+ YOUR AIMS
- To control blood loss and minimise the effects of shock.
- To minimise the risk of infection.
- To arrange transport to hospital.

1 Put on disposable gloves if available. Press a sterile wound dressing or clean pad firmly into the palm, and ask the casualty to clench his fist over it. If he cannot press hard, tell him to grasp his fist with his uninjured hand.

2 Bandage the casualty's fingers so that they are clenched over the pad. Tie the ends of the bandage over the top of the fingers.

Leave thumb free

Raise and support arm

3 Support the casualty's arm in an elevation sling (p.18) to keep it raised. Arrange to take or send the casualty to hospital.

WOUND AT A JOINT CREASE

Major blood vessels inside the elbows and knees will bleed copiously if severed. The steps below help control bleeding and shock; but because they also impede blood flow to the lower part of the limb, you must keep checking circulation to this area.

▶ See also FOREIGN OBJECT IN A CUT p.63
● SHOCK pp.50–51

+ YOUR AIMS
- To control blood loss and minimise the effects of shock.
- To minimise the risk of infection.
- To arrange transport to hospital.

1 Put on disposable gloves if available. Press a sterile wound dressing or clean pad on the injury. Bend the joint to hold the pad and keep pressure on the wound.

2 Raise and support the limb. If possible, help the casualty lie down with his legs raised and supported.

3 Take or send the casualty to hospital in the final treatment position. Every 10 minutes, check the circulation beyond the injury. If necessary, briefly release the pressure on the wound to restore normal blood flow to the lower part of the limb, then reapply pressure.

5

THE SKELETON is the supporting framework around which the body is constructed. It is jointed in many places, and muscles attached to the bones enable us to move. Most of our movements are controlled at will and coordinated by impulses that travel from the brain via the nerves to every muscle and joint in the body.

DIAGNOSING TYPES OF INJURY
Because it is sometimes difficult to distinguish between bone, joint, and muscle injuries, the chapter begins with an overview of the types of injury. First-aid treatments for most injuries, from major fractures to sprains and dislocations, are given here. Skull fracture is covered in the chapter on disorders of consciousness (p.90) because of the potential damage to the brain that this injury can cause.

CONTENTS

Types of injury..........................70

Strains and sprains..................72

Cheekbone and nose
    fractures 73

Fractured collar bone 74

Shoulder injury........................75

Arm injury................................76

Elbow injury.............................77

Hand and finger injuries..........78

Spinal injury 79

Fractured pelvis 82

Hip and thigh injuries..............83

Knee injury 84

Lower leg injury ,,,,,,,.............85

Ankle injury 86

Foot and toe injuries. 86

BONE, JOINT, AND MUSCLE INJURIES

+ FIRST-AID PRIORITIES

- Assess the casualty's condition.
- Comfort and reassure the casualty.
- Steady and support the injured part.
- Enhance the support with padding, bandages, and splints if necessary.
- Minimise shock.
- Obtain medical aid if necessary. Call an ambulance if you suspect a serious injury.

TYPES OF INJURY

A break or crack in a bone is known as a fracture. Bones are not brittle like chalk, but tough and resilient. When struck or twisted, they bend like branches. This means that generally, considerable force is needed to break a bone, unless it is diseased or old. Growing bones, however, are supple and may split, bend, or crack.

A joint may become dislocated, with the bones being partially or completely pulled out of position. Dislocation can result from the bone being wrenched into an abnormal position or violent muscle contraction.

Strains and sprains result from injury to, or overstretching of, the muscles, ligaments, or tendons.

FRACTURES

A bone may break at the point where a heavy blow is received – for example, when struck by a car (direct force). Fractures may also result from a twist or a wrench (indirect force).

STABLE AND UNSTABLE FRACTURES
In a stable fracture, the broken bone ends do not move because they are incompletely broken or jammed together. Usually, they can be gently treated without causing more damage.

In an unstable fracture, the broken bone ends can easily move out of position. As a result, there is a risk that they may damage blood vessels, nerves, and organs. Unstable injuries

can occur if the bone is completely broken or the ligaments are torn (ruptured). Handle these injuries very carefully to avoid further damage.

OPEN AND CLOSED FRACTURES
In an open fracture, one of the broken bone ends may pierce the skin surface, or there may be a wound at the fracture site, carrying a high risk of infection.

In a closed fracture, the skin above the fracture is intact. However, bones may be displaced (unstable) and damage internal tissues. If the bone ends pierce organs or major blood vessels, the casualty may have internal bleeding and suffer shock (pp.50–51).

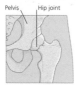

Pelvis   Hip joint

Stable injury
Although the bone is fractured, the ends of the injury remain in place. The risk of bleeding or further damage is minimal.

Thigh bone

Unstable injury
In this type of fracture, the broken bone ends can easily be displaced by movement or muscle contraction, which can lead to further damage.

Closed fracture
The skin is not broken, although the bone ends may damage nearby tissues and blood vessels. Internal bleeding is a risk.

Open fracture
Bone is exposed at the surface where it breaks the skin. The casualty is likely to suffer bleeding and shock. Infection is a risk.

DISLOCATIONS

These very painful injuries often affect the shoulder (see SHOULDER INJURY, p.74), jaw, or joints in the thumbs or fingers. Dislocations may be associated with torn ligaments (see below) or damage to the synovial membrane, which lines the joint capsule.

In some cases, joint dislocation can be serious. Dislocation of the shoulder or hip may damage major nerves that supply the limbs and result in paralysis. A severe dislocation of any joint may also fracture the bones involved.

It can be difficult to distinguish a dislocation from a closed fracture. If in doubt, treat the injury as a fracture.

MUSCLE, TENDON, AND LIGAMENT INJURIES

The softer structures around bones and joints – the ligaments, muscles, and tendons – may be injured in several ways. Injuries to these soft tissues are commonly called strains and sprains (p.72). They occur when the tissues are overstretched and partially or completely torn (ruptured) by violent or sudden movements.

LIGAMENT INJURY

Ligaments connect bones at a joint. They may become torn due to a sudden or unexpected wrenching that pulls the bones in the joint too far apart and tears the surrounding tissues.

Sprained ankle

This is due to overstretching or tearing of a ligament – the fibrous cords that connect bones at a joint. In this example, one of the ligaments in the ankle is partially torn.

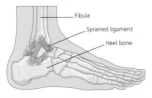

Fibula

Sprained ligament

Heel bone

MUSCLE AND TENDON INJURY

Muscles and tendons (which attach muscle to bone) may be strained, ruptured, or bruised. A strain often occurs at the point where the tendon attaches to the bone. In a rupture, a muscle or tendon is torn completely; this may occur in the main bulk of the muscle or in the tendon.

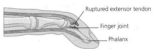

Ruptured extensor tendon

Finger joint

Phalanx

Torn finger tendon

Tendons attach muscle to bone across a joint. If a hard object strikes the end of the finger, the extensor tendon, which passes over the top of the finger joint, may be torn from its attachment.

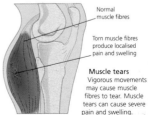

Normal muscle fibres

Torn muscle fibres produce localised pain and swelling

Muscle tears

Vigorous movements may cause muscle fibres to tear. Muscle tears can cause severe pain and swelling.

STRAINS AND SPRAINS

Ligaments, muscles, and tendons can be overstretched and partially or completely torn (ruptured) by violent or sudden movements. Deep bruising may be extensive in parts of the body where there is a large bulk of muscle. Such injuries are usually accompanied by bleeding into surrounding tissues, which can lead to pain, swelling, and bruising. Follow the "RICE" procedure to treat sprains and strains:
R – *Rest* the injured part.
I – Apply *Ice* or a cold compress.

C – *Compress* the injury.
E – *Elevate* the injured part.
If you are in any doubt as to the severity of the injury, arrange to take or send the casualty to hospital.

+ YOUR AIMS
● To reduce swelling and pain.
● To obtain medical aid if necessary.

1 Advise the casualty to sit or lie down. Support the injured part in a comfortable position.

Use your knee to support injured leg

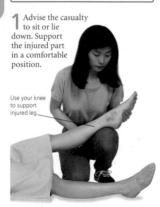

2 If the injury has just happened, cool the area by applying an ice pack or cold pad (p.12). This will help to reduce swelling, bruising, and pain.

3 Apply gentle, even pressure (compression) to the injured part by surrounding the area with a thick layer of soft padding, such as cotton wool or plastic foam, and securing this layer of padding with a bandage. Check the circulation beyond the bandaging (p.14) every 10 minutes.

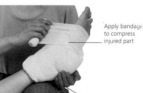

Apply bandage to compress injured part

Support foot

4 Raise (elevate) and support the injured part to reduce the flow of blood to the injury. This action will help to minimise bruising in the area.

5 If the pain is severe, or the casualty is unable to use the injured part, take or send the casualty to hospital. Otherwise, advise the casualty to rest and to see her doctor if necessary.

CHEEKBONE & NOSE FRACTURES

Fractures of the cheekbone and nose are usually the result of deliberate blows to the face. Swollen facial tissues are likely to cause discomfort, and the air passages in the nose may become blocked, making breathing difficult. These injuries should always be examined in hospital.

> See also NOSEBLEED p.66

RECOGNITION

There may be:
- Pain, swelling, and bruising.
- A wound or bleeding from the nose or mouth.

+ YOUR AIMS

- To minimise pain and swelling.
- To arrange to transport or send the casualty to hospital.

❶ CAUTION

If there is straw-coloured fluid leaking from the casualty's nose, treat the casualty as for a skull fracture (p.90).

1 Gently apply a cold compress (p.12) to the injured area to help reduce pain and limit potential swelling.

2 If the casualty has a nosebleed, try to stop the bleeding (p.66). Arrange to transport or send the casualty to hospital.

LOWER JAW INJURY

Jaw fractures are usually the result of direct force, such as a heavy blow to the chin. In some cases, a blow to one side of the jaw may cause a fracture on the other side. A fall on to the point of the chin can fracture the jaw on both sides. The lower jaw may also be dislocated by a blow to the face, or is sometimes dislocated by yawning.

RECOGNITION

There may be:
- Difficulty speaking, swallowing, and moving the jaw.
- Pain and nausea when moving the jaw.
- Displaced or loose teeth and dribbling.
- Swelling and bruising inside and outside the mouth.

+ YOUR AIMS

- To protect the airway.
- To arrange transport to hospital.

❶ CAUTION

Do not bandage padding in case the casualty vomits or has difficulty breathing.

1 If the casualty is not seriously injured, help him to sit with his head well forward to allow fluids to drain from his mouth. Encourage the casualty to spit out loose teeth, and keep them to send to hospital with him.

2 Give the casualty a soft pad to hold firmly against his jaw in order to support it.

3 Take or send the casualty to hospital, keeping his jaw supported.

FRACTURED COLLAR BONE

It is rare for a collar bone to be broken by a direct blow. Usually, a fracture results from an indirect force as a result of impact at the shoulder or passing along the arm, for example from a fall on to an outstretched arm. These injuries often occur in young people as a result of sports activities. The broken ends of the collar bone may be displaced, causing swelling and bleeding in the surrounding tissues, and distortion of the shoulder.

RECOGNITION

There may be:
• Pain and tenderness, increased by movement.
• Swelling and deformity of the shoulder.
• Attempts by the casualty to relax muscles and relieve pain; she may support the arm at the elbow, and incline the head to the injured side.

See also FRACTURES p.70

✚ YOUR AIMS

• To immobilise the injured upper limb.
• To arrange transport to hospital.

1 Help the casualty to sit down. Lay the affected arm diagonally across her chest with her fingertips resting against the opposite shoulder. Ask her to support the elbow with her other hand.

3 Carefully place some soft padding, such as a small towel or folded clothing, between the arm and the body to make the casualty more comfortable.

4 Secure the arm to the chest with a broad-fold bandage (p.16) tied around the chest and over the sling.

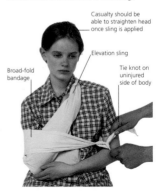

Injury makes casualty incline head to injured side

Remove any restricting clothing, such as a bra strap, if it is causing discomfort

Ask casualty to support elbow

Casualty should be able to straighten head once sling is applied

Broad-fold bandage

Elevation sling

Tie knot on uninjured side of body

2 Support the arm on the affected side in an elevation sling (p.18).

5 Arrange to take or send the casualty to hospital in a sitting position.

SHOULDER INJURY

A fall on to the shoulder or an outstretched arm, or a wrenching force, may pull the head of the arm bone (humerus) out of the joint socket. Ligaments around the shoulder joint may also be torn. This painful injury is called dislocation of the shoulder and requires hospital treatment.

A fall on to the point of the shoulder may damage the ligaments bracing the collar bone at the shoulder. Other shoulder injuries include damage to the joint capsule and to the tendons around the shoulder; these injuries tend to be common in older people and should be treated by following the RICE procedure (p.72).

▶ See also SPRAINS AND STRAINS p.72

YOUR AIMS

• To support the injured limb.
• To arrange urgent removal to hospital.

CAUTION

• Do not attempt to replace a dislocated bone into its socket.
• Do not allow the casualty to eat, drink, or smoke because a general anaesthetic may be necessary in hospital.

1 Help the casualty to sit down. Gently place the arm on the affected side across her body in the position that is most comfortable.

2 Place a triangular bandage between the arm and the chest, in preparation for tying an arm sling (p.17).

3 Insert soft padding, such as a folded towel or clothing, between the arm and the chest, inside the bandage.

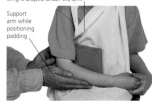

Sling is draped under the arm

Support arm while positioning padding

4 Finish tying the arm sling so that the arm and its padding are well supported.

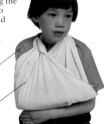

Site of injury

Keep bandage clear of injury site

5 Secure the limb to the chest by tying a broad-fold bandage (p.16) around the chest and over the sling.

6 Arrange to take or send the casualty to hospital in a sitting position.

ARM INJURY

The most serious form of upper arm injury is a fracture of the long bone in the upper arm (humerus). It is common, especially in elderly people, for the arm bone to break at the shoulder end, usually in a fall.

The bones of the forearm (radius and ulna) can be fractured by an impact such as a heavy blow or a fall on to an outstretched hand. As the bones have little fleshy covering, the broken ends may pierce the skin, producing an open fracture (p.70).

At the wrist, the most common form of fracture is a Colles' fracture, which is a break at the end of the radius. This injury often occurs in older women. In a young adult, a fall may break one of the small wrist bones (carpals).

> See also ELBOW INJURY opposite

See also ELBOW INJURY opposite

RECOGNITION

There may be:
- Pain, increased by movement.
- Tenderness and deformity over the site of a fracture.
- Swelling and bruising.

YOUR AIMS

- To immobilise the arm.
- To arrange transport to hospital.

1 Ask the casualty to sit down. Steady and support the forearm by placing it across his body. Expose and treat any wound you find, wearing disposable gloves if available.

2 Place a triangular bandage between the chest and the injured arm, as for an arm sling (p.17). Surround the forearm in soft padding, such as a small towel or a thick layer of cotton wool.

3 Fasten the sling around the arm and its padding using a reef knot (p.16). Tie the knot at the hollow of the casualty's collar bone on the injured side.

4 If the journey to hospital is likely to be prolonged, secure the arm to the body by tying a broad-fold bandage (p.16) over the sling, positioning it close to the elbow. Then take or send the casualty to hospital.

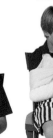

Cradle arm in folds of soft padding

Ask casualty to support injured arm

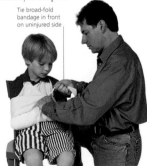

Tie broad-fold bandage in front on uninjured side

ELBOW INJURY

Fractures or dislocations at the elbow usually result from a fall on to the hand. This is an unstable fracture (p.70), and the bone ends may damage blood vessels. Circulation in the arm needs to be checked regularly. In any elbow injury, the elbow will be stiff and difficult to straighten. Never try to force it to bend.

RECOGNITION

There may be:

- Pain, increased by movement.
- Tenderness over the site of a fracture.
- Swelling, bruising, and deformity.
- Fixed elbow.

▶ See also ARM INJURY opposite

FOR AN ELBOW THAT CAN BEND

+ YOUR AIMS

- To immobilise the arm without further injury to the joint.
- To arrange transport to hospital.

▶ Treat as for ARM INJURY opposite

❶ CAUTION

Check the pulse in the affected wrist regularly (p.8). If the pulse is not present, gently straighten the elbow until the pulse returns. Support the arm in this position.

FOR AN ELBOW THAT CANNOT BEND

+ YOUR AIMS

- To immobilise the arm without further injury to the joint.
- To arrange transport to hospital.

❶ WARNING

- Do not try to move the injured arm.
- Do not attempt to apply bandages if help is on its way.

1 Help the casualty to lie down. Place padding, such as towels, around the elbow for comfort and support.

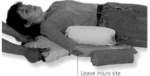

Leave injury site free of padding

2 DIAL 999 FOR AN AMBULANCE Check the pulse (p.8) in the injured arm until medical help arrives.

SPECIAL CASE

PREPARING FOR TRANSPORT
Put padding between the injured limb and body. Then use three folded triangular bandages to immobilise the injured limb against the trunk, at the wrist and hips (1), then above (2) and below (3) the elbow.

Tie bandages firmly on the non-injured side

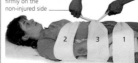

HAND AND FINGER INJURIES

Minor fractures of the bones or joints in the hand are usually caused by direct force. The most common type – a fracture of the knuckle between the little finger and the hand – often results from a misdirected punch.

Multiple fractures are usually caused by crushing injuries. The fractures may be open, with severe bleeding and swelling, needing immediate first-aid treatment.

The joints in the fingers or thumb are sometimes dislocated or sprained as a result of a fall on to the hand.

> RECOGNITION

There may be:
- Pain, increased by movement.
- Swelling, bruising, and deformity.
- In an open fracture, a wound and bleeding.

Always compare a suspected fractured hand with the normal hand because finger fractures result in deformities that may not be immediately obvious.

▶ See also DISLOCATED JOINT p.71 ● FRACTURES p.70 ● WOUND TO THE PALM p.68

> ✛ YOUR AIMS
> - To immobilise and elevate the hand.
> - To arrange transport to hospital.

1 If there is any bleeding, put on disposable gloves, if available. Apply a clean, non-fluffy dressing to the wound.

2 Remove any rings before the hand begins to swell, and then keep the hand raised to reduce swelling. Protect the injured area by wrapping the hand in folds of soft padding.

3 Gently support the affected arm across the casualty's body by applying an elevation sling (p.18).

4 If necessary, secure the arm to the casualty's body by tying a broad-fold bandage (p.16) around the chest and over the sling. Then arrange to take or send the casualty to hospital.

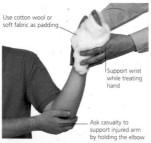

Use cotton wool or soft fabric as padding

Support wrist while treating hand

Ask casualty to support injured arm by holding the elbow

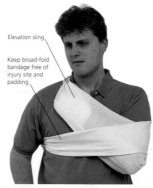

Elevation sling

Keep broad-fold bandage free of injury site and padding

SPINAL INJURY

Injuries to the spine can involve one or more parts of the back and/or neck: the bones (vertebrae), the discs of tissue that separate the vertebrae, the surrounding muscles and ligaments, or the spinal cord and the nerves that branch off from it.

The most serious risk associated with spinal injury is damage to the spinal cord. Such damage can cause loss of power and/or sensation below the injured area. The spinal cord or nerve roots can suffer temporary damage if they are pinched by displaced or dislocated discs or by fragments of broken bone. If the cord is partly or completely severed, the damage may be permanent.

WHEN TO SUSPECT SPINAL INJURY
The most important indicator is the mechanism of the injury. Always suspect spinal injury if abnormal forces have been exerted on the back or neck, and particularly if the casualty complains of any interference with feeling or movement. Take care to avoid unnecessary movement of the head and neck at all times.

SOME CAUSES OF SPINAL INJURY
Any of the following circumstances should alert you to a possible spinal injury:
- Falling from a height.
- Falling awkwardly while doing gymnastics or trampolining.
- Diving into a shallow pool and hitting the bottom.
- Being thrown from a horse or motorbike.
- Being in a collapsed rugby scrum.
- Sudden deceleration in a vehicle.
- A heavy object falling across the back.
- Injury to the head or the face.

Continued on next page

RECOGNITION

When the vertebrae are damaged, there may be:
- Pain in the neck or back at the injury site; this may be masked by other, more painful injuries.
- A step, irregularity, or twist in the normal curve of the spine.
- Tenderness in the skin over the spine.

When the spinal cord is damaged, there may be:
- Loss of control over limbs; movement may be weak or absent.
- Loss of sensation, or abnormal sensations such as burning or tingling. The casualty may say that limbs feel stiff, heavy, or clumsy.
- Loss of bladder and/or bowel control.
- Breathing difficulties.

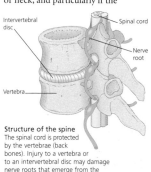

Intervertebral disc

Spinal cord

Nerve root

Vertebra

Structure of the spine
The spinal cord is protected by the vertebrae (back bones). Injury to a vertebra or to an intervertebral disc may damage nerve roots that emerge from the spinal cord or damage the cord itself.

SPINAL INJURY (continued)

FOR A CONSCIOUS CASUALTY

+ YOUR AIMS

- To prevent further injury.
- To arrange urgent removal to hospital.

! CAUTION

- Do not move the casualty from the position in which you found her unless she is in danger.
- If the casualty has to be moved, use the log-roll technique (opposite). Alternatively, use an orthopaedic stretcher.

1 Reassure the casualty and advise her not to move.
DIAL 999 FOR AN AMBULANCE

2 Kneel behind the casualty's head. Grasp the sides of the casualty's head firmly, with your hands over the ears. Do not completely cover her ears – she should still be able to hear you. Steady and support her head in the neutral position, in which the head, neck, and spine are aligned. This is the least harmful head position for a casualty with a suspected spinal injury.

Rest arms on legs to keep them steady

Hold casualty's head straight to steady the neck, but do not completely cover her ears

! WARNING

If you suspect neck injury, ask a helper to place rolled-up blankets, towels, or items of clothing on either side of the casualty's head and neck, while you keep her head in the neutral position.

Continue to support the casualty's head and neck throughout until emergency medical services take over.

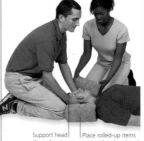

Support head throughout | Place rolled-up items against head and neck

3 Continue to support the casualty's head in the neutral position until emergency medical services take over, no matter how long this may be. Get help to monitor and record her vital signs – level of response, pulse, and breathing (pp.8–9).

FOR AN UNCONSCIOUS CASUALTY

- To maintain an open airway.
- To resuscitate the casualty if necessary.
- To prevent further spinal damage.
- To arrange urgent removal to hospital.

1 Kneel behind the casualty's head. Grasp the sides of her head firmly with your hands over the ears. Steady and support her head in the neutral head position, in which the head, neck, and spine are aligned.

2 If necessary, open the casualty's airway using the jaw thrust method. Place your hands on each side of her face with your fingertips at the angles of the jaw. Gently lift her jaw to open the airway. Take care not to tilt the casualty's neck.

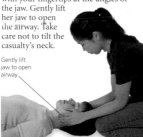

Gently lift jaw to open airway

3 Check the casualty's breathing. If she is breathing, continue to support her head. Ask a helper to DIAL 999 FOR AN AMBULANCE. If you are alone and you need to leave the casualty to call an ambulance, and if the casualty is unable to maintain an open airway, you should turn her into the recovery position (pp.30–31) before you leave her.

SPECIAL CASE

LOG-ROLL TECHNIQUE
This technique should be used if you have to turn a casualty with a spinal injury. Ideally, you need five helpers but the move can be done with three. While you support the casualty's head and neck, ask your helpers to straighten her limbs gently. Then, ensuring that everyone works together, direct your helpers to roll the casualty. Keep the casualty's head, trunk, and toes in a straight line at all times.

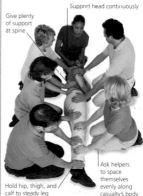

Give plenty of support at spine

Support head continuously

Ask helpers to space themselves evenly along casualty's body

Hold hip, thigh, and calf to steady leg

4 If the casualty is not breathing, and there are no signs of circulation, give rescue breaths and chest compressions (see LIFE-SAVING PROCEDURES, pp.19–48). If you have to turn the casualty, use the log-roll technique (above).

5 Monitor and record vital signs – level of response, pulse, and breathing (pp.8–9) – until medical help arrives.

FRACTURED PELVIS

Injuries to the pelvis are usually caused by indirect force, such as in a car crash or by crushing. For example, the impact of a car dashboard on a knee can force the head of the thigh bone through the hip socket.

A fracture of the pelvic bones may be complicated by injury to tissues and organs inside the pelvis, such as the bladder. In addition, internal bleeding may be severe because there are major organs and blood vessels in the pelvis. Shock often develops as a result, and should be treated promptly.

RECOGNITION

There may be:
● Inability to walk or even stand, although the legs appear uninjured.
● Pain and tenderness in the region of the hip, groin, or back, which increases with movement.
● Blood at the urinary outlet, especially in a male casualty. The casualty may not be able to pass urine or may find this painful.
● Signs of shock and internal bleeding.

▶ See also SHOCK pp.50–51

✚ YOUR AIMS

● To minimise the risk of shock.
● To arrange urgent removal to hospital.

❶ CAUTION

Do not bandage the casualty's legs together if this causes any more pain. In such cases, surround the injured area with soft padding such as clothing or towels.

1 Help the casualty to lie down on his back. Keep his legs straight and flat or, if it is more comfortable, help him to bend his knees slightly and support them with padding, such as a cushion or folded clothing.

2 Place padding between the bony points of the knees and the ankles. Immobilise the legs by bandaging them together with folded triangular bandages; secure the feet and ankles (1), then the knees (2).

3 DIAL 999 FOR AN AMBULANCE. Treat the casualty for shock (pp.50–51).

4 Monitor and record vital signs – level of response, breathing, and pulse (pp.8–9) – until help arrives.

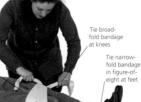

Tie broad-fold bandage at knees

Tie narrow-fold bandage in figure-of-eight at feet

Place soft padding between knees

Keep head flat to minimise shock

HIP AND THIGH INJURIES

The most serious injury of the thigh bone (femur) is a fracture. It takes a considerable force, such as a traffic incident or a fall from a height, to fracture the shaft of the femur. This is a serious injury because the broken bone ends can pierce major blood vessels, causing heavy blood loss, and shock (pp.50–51) may result.

In the hip joint, the most serious, though much less common, type of injury is dislocation.

● See also DISLOCATED JOINT p.71
● FRACTURES p.70 ● SHOCK pp.50–51

RECOGNITION

There may be:
● Pain at the site of the injury.
● Inability to walk.
● Signs of shock.
● Shortening of the leg and turning outwards of the knee and foot, as powerful muscles move the broken bone ends over each other.

+ YOUR AIMS

● To immobilise the lower limb.
● To arrange urgent removal to hospital.

! WARNING

● Do not allow the casualty to eat, drink, or smoke, because he may need to have a general anaesthetic in hospital.
● Do not raise the casualty's legs, even if he shows any signs of shock, because you may cause further internal damage.

1 Help the casualty to lie down. If possible, ask a helper to gently steady and support the injured limb. Gently straighten his lower leg.

2 DIAL 999 FOR AN AMBULANCE
If the ambulance is expected to arrive quickly, support the leg in the same position until the ambulance arrives.

3 If the ambulance is not expected to arrive quickly, immobilise the leg by splinting it to the uninjured one. Gently bring the sound limb alongside the injured one. Position bandages at the ankles and feet (1), then the knees (2). Add bandages above (3) and below (4) the fracture site. Insert soft padding between the legs to prevent the bony parts from rubbing against each other, then tie the bandages on the uninjured side.

4 Treat the casualty for shock (pp.50–51): insulate him from the cold with blankets or clothing, but do not raise his legs.

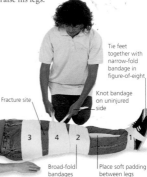

Tie feet together with narrow-fold bandage in figure-of-eight

Knot bandage on uninjured side

Fracture site

Broad-fold bandages

Place soft padding between legs

KNEE INJURY

The knee is the hinge joint between the thigh bone (femur) and shin bone (tibia). The knee is supported by strong muscles and ligaments and protected at the front by a disc of bone called the kneecap (patella). Discs of cartilage protect the surfaces of the major bones. These structures may be damaged by direct blows, violent twists, or sprains. Possible knee injuries include fracture of the patella, sprains, and damage to the cartilage.

The casualty may be unable to bend an injured knee joint; you should

| RECOGNITION |

There may be:
- Pain, spreading from the injury to become deep-seated in the joint.
- If the bent knee has "locked", acute pain on attempting to straighten the leg.
- Rapid swelling at the knee joint.

ensure that the casualty does not try to walk on the injured leg.

Bleeding or fluid in the knee joint may cause swelling around the knee.

▶ See also SPRAINS AND STRAINS p.72

| YOUR AIMS |

- To protect the knee in the most comfortable position.
- To arrange removal to hospital.

| WARNING |

- Do not attempt to straighten the knee forcibly. Displaced cartilage or internal bleeding may make it impossible to straighten the knee joint safely.
- Do not allow the casualty to eat, drink, or smoke, because she may need a general anaesthetic in hospital.
- Do not allow the casualty to walk.

1 Help the casualty to lie down, preferably on a blanket to insulate her from the ground. Place soft padding, such as a pillow, blanket, or coat, under her injured knee to support it in the most comfortable position.

2 Wrap padding around the joint and secure with bandages that extend from mid-thigh to the middle of the lower leg.

3 Arrange removal of the casualty to hospital. The casualty needs to remain in the treatment position and so should be transported in an ambulance.

Use roller bandage to hold padding in place

Support casualty's knee with soft padding

LOWER LEG INJURY

Injuries to the lower leg include fractures of the shin bone (tibia) and the splint bone (fibula), and tearing of the soft tissues. Fractures of the tibia are usually due to a heavy blow and are likely to produce a wound. The fibula can be broken by the twisting that sprains an ankle.

See also SPRAINS AND STRAINS p.72

RECOGNITION

There may be:
- Localised pain.
- Swelling, bruising, and deformity of the leg.
- An open wound.

YOUR AIMS

- To immobilise the leg.
- To arrange urgent removal to hospital.

1 Help the casualty to lie down, and carefully steady and support the injured leg. If there is an open wound, gently expose the wound and treat bleeding. Apply padding to protect the injury.

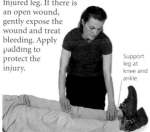

Support leg at knee and ankle

2 DIAL 999 FOR AN AMBULANCE Support the injured leg with your hands to prevent any movement of the fracture site. Maintain this support until the ambulance arrives.

⚠ CAUTION

If the casualty's journey to hospital is likely to be long and rough, place soft padding on the outside of the injured leg, from the knee to the foot. Secure legs with broad-fold bandages as described above.

3 If the ambulance is delayed, support the injured leg by splinting it to the other leg. Bring the uninjured limb alongside the injured one and slide bandages under both legs. Place bandages at the feet and ankles (1), then knees (2). Add bandages above (3) and below (4) the fracture. Insert padding between the lower legs. Then tie the bandages firmly, knotting them on the uninjured side.

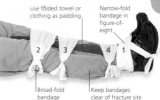

Use folded towel or clothing as padding

Narrow-fold bandage in figure-of-eight

Broad-fold bandage

Keep bandages clear of fracture site

SPECIAL CASE

SUSPECTED FRACTURE NEAR ANKLE
Place separate bandages above the ankle and around the feet, rather than one figure-of-eight.

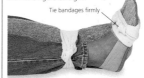

Tie bandages firmly

ANKLE INJURY

If the ankle is broken, treat it as a fracture of the lower leg (p.85). A more common injury is a sprain (p.72), which can be treated with the RICE procedure: *Rest* the affected part, apply *Ice*, *Compress* with bandaging, and *Elevate* (below).

▶ See also SPRAINS AND STRAINS p.72

RECOGNITION
- Pain, increased either by movement or by putting weight on the foot.
- Swelling.

+ YOUR AIMS
- To relieve pain and swelling.
- To obtain medical aid if necessary.

! CAUTION
If you suspect a broken bone, tell the casualty not to put weight on the leg. Secure and support the lower leg (p.85), and take or send the casualty to hospital.

1 Rest, steady, and support the ankle in the most comfortable position.

2 If the injury has occurred recently, apply an ice pack or a cold compress (p.12) to the site to reduce swelling.

3 Wrap the ankle in thick padding and bandage firmly. Raise and support the limb. Advise the casualty to rest the ankle and to see a doctor if pain persists.

FOOT AND TOE INJURIES

Fractures affecting the bones of the foot are usually caused by crushing. They are best treated in hospital. When giving first aid, concentrate on relieving symptoms such as swelling.

RECOGNITION
- Difficulty in walking.
- Stiffness of movement.
- Bruising and swelling.

+ YOUR AIMS
- To minimise swelling.
- To arrange transport to hospital.

1 Quickly raise and support the foot to minimise swelling.

2 Apply an ice pack or cold compress (p.12) to relieve swelling.

3 Arrange for the casualty to go to hospital. Ensure the foot remains elevated during the journey.

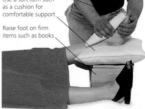

Apply ice pack to reduce swelling

Use a soft item such as a cushion for comfortable support

Raise foot on firm items such as books

6

THE NERVOUS SYSTEM is the most complex system in the body. Its control centre, the brain, is the source of consciousness, thought, speech, and memory. The brain also receives and interprets sensory information, which is carried by the nerves, and controls other body systems. If consciousness is impaired, even survival mechanisms, such as the cough reflex to keep the airway clear, may not function

TREATMENT PRIORITIES
Because the problems described in this chapter can produce impaired consciousness, they need immediate attention. Your first-aid priorities are to monitor and maintain the vital functions of breathing and circulation and get medical help if necessary.

FIRST-AID PRIORITIES

- Assess the casualty's condition.
- Comfort and reassure the casualty.
- Maintain an open airway, check breathing, and be prepared to resuscitate if necessary.
- Protect the casualty from harm.
- Look for and treat any injuries associated with the condition.
- Obtain medical aid if necessary. Call an ambulance if you suspect a serious illness or injury.

CONTENTS

Concussion 88

Cerebral compression..............89

Skull fracture 90

Stroke....................................91

Diabetes mellitus....................92

Hyperglycaemia......................92

Hypoglycaemia.......................93

Seizures in adults 94

Absence seizures....................95

Seizures in children 96

DISORDERS OF CONSCIOUSNESS

CONCUSSION

The brain moves a little within the skull and it can be "shaken" by a blow to the head, which is known as concussion. Common causes include traffic incidents, sports injuries, and falls. Concussion produces widespread temporary disturbance of normal brain activity but is not usually associated with any lasting damage to the brain. The casualty will suffer impaired consciousness, but this usually lasts for only a few minutes and is followed by a full recovery.

A casualty who has been concussed should be monitored and advised to obtain medical aid immediately should symptoms such as headache or blurred vision develop later.

▶ See also CEREBRAL COMPRESSION pp.89
● LIFE-SAVING PROCEDURES pp.19–48
● SPINAL INJURY pp.79–81

RECOGNITION

● Brief period of impaired consciousness following a blow to the head.
There may also be:
● Dizziness or nausea on recovery.
● Loss of memory of events at the time of, or immediately preceding, the injury.
● Mild, generalised headache.

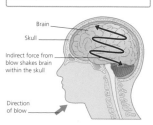

Brain
Skull
Indirect force from blow shakes brain within the skull
Direction of blow

Mechanism of concussion
Concussion usually occurs as a result of a blow to the head. This "shakes" the brain within the skull, causing brain function to be disturbed temporarily.

✚ YOUR AIMS

● To ensure the casualty recovers safely.
● To place the casualty in the care of a responsible person.
● To obtain medical aid if necessary.

❶ WARNING

If the casualty does not recover fully, OR if there is a deteriorating level of response after an initial recovery
DIAL 999 FOR AN AMBULANCE

❶ CAUTION

All casualties who have had a head injury should also be treated for a neck injury (see SPINAL INJURY, pp.79–81).

1 Perform a check of consciousness following the APVU code (p.8).

2 Monitor and record vital signs – level of response, pulse, and breathing (pp.8–9). Even if the casualty appears to recover, watch him for subsequent deterioration in his level of response.

3 When the casualty has recovered, place him in the care of a responsible person. If he has been injured on the sports field, never allow him to "play on" without first obtaining medical advice.

4 Advise the casualty to go to hospital if he later develops symptoms such as headache, nausea, vomiting, or excessive sleepiness following a blow to the head.

CEREBRAL COMPRESSION

Compression of the brain, or cerebral compression, is very serious and almost invariably requires surgery. Cerebral compression occurs when there is a build-up of pressure on the brain. This pressure may be due to one of several different causes, such as an accumulation of blood within the skull or swelling of injured brain tissues.

Cerebral compression is usually caused by a head injury. However, it can also be due to other causes, such as a stroke (p.91), infection, or brain tumour. The condition may develop immediately after a head injury, or it may appear a few hours or even days later. For this reason, try to find out whether the casualty has a recent history of a head injury.

⊙ See also LIFE-SAVING PROCEDURES pp.19–48 • SPINAL INJURY pp.79–81

Compression caused by bleeding
Bleeding may occur within the skull following a head injury or a disorder such as a stroke. The escaped blood may put pressure on brain tissues.

RECOGNITION

• Deteriorating level of response – casualty may become unconscious.
There may also be:
• History of a recent head injury.
• Intense headache.
• Noisy breathing, becoming slow.
• Slow, yet full and strong pulse.
• Unequal pupil size.
• Weakness and/or paralysis down one side of the face or body.
• High temperature; flushed face.
• Drowsiness.
• Change in personality or behaviour, such as irritability or disorientation.

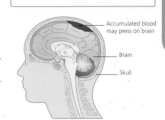

Accumulated blood may press on brain

Brain

Skull

✚ YOUR AIM

• To arrange urgent removal of the casualty to hospital.

ⓘ WARNING

If the casualty is unconscious, open the airway using the jaw thrust method (p.81) and check breathing; be prepared to give rescue breaths and chest compressions (*see* LIFE-SAVING PROCEDURES, pp.19–48).
DIAL 999 FOR AN AMBULANCE
If breathing, try to maintain the airway in the position the casualty was found.

1 **DIAL 999 FOR AN AMBULANCE**
If the casualty is conscious, try to keep him supported in a comfortable resting position and reassure him.

2 Monitor and record the casualty's vital signs – level of response, pulse, and breathing (pp.8–9) –regularly until medical help arrives.

ⓘ CAUTION

Do not allow the casualty to eat, drink, or smoke because a general anaesthetic may need to be given in hospital.

SKULL FRACTURE

A skull fracture is very serious because there is a risk that the brain may be damaged either directly by fractured bone from the skull or by bleeding inside the skull. Clear fluid (cerebrospinal fluid) or watery blood leaking from the ear or nose are signs of serious injury.

You should suspect a skull fracture in any casualty who has received a head injury resulting in impaired consciousness. Bear in mind that a casualty with a possible skull fracture may also have a neck (spinal) injury and should be treated accordingly (see SPINAL INJURY, pp.79–81).

RECOGNITION

- Wound or bruise on the head.
- Soft area or depression on the scalp.
- Bruising or swelling behind one ear.
- Bruising around one or both eyes.
- Clear fluid or watery blood coming from the nose or an ear.
- Blood in the white of the eye.
- Distortion or lack of symmetry of the head and face.
- Progressive deterioration in the level of response.

▶ See also LIFE-SAVING PROCEDURES pp.19–48 ● SCALP AND HEAD WOUNDS p.64 ● SPINAL INJURY pp.79–81

➕ YOUR AIMS

- To maintain an open airway.
- To arrange urgent removal of the casualty to hospital.

1 If the casualty is conscious, help her to lie down. Do not turn the head in case there is a neck injury.

2 Control any bleeding from the scalp by applying pressure around the wound. Look for and treat any other injuries.
DIAL 999 FOR AN AMBULANCE

3 If there is discharge from an ear, cover the ear with a sterile dressing or clean pad, lightly secured with a bandage (see BLEEDING FROM THE EAR, p.65). Do not plug the ear.

4 Regularly monitor and record vital signs – level of response, pulse, and breathing (pp.8–9) – until medical help arrives.

❶ WARNING

If the casualty is unconscious, open the airway using the jaw thrust method (p.81) and check breathing; be ready to give rescue breaths and chest compressions if needed (see LIFE-SAVING PROCEDURES, pp.19–48).
DIAL 999 FOR AN AMBULANCE

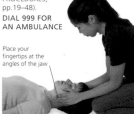

Place your fingertips at the angles of the jaw

If the position in which the casualty was found prevents maintenance of an open airway or you fail to open it using the jaw thrust, place her in the recovery position (pp.30–31). If you have helpers, use the "log-roll" technique (p.81).

STROKE

A "stroke" is a condition in which the blood supply to part of the brain is suddenly and seriously impaired by a blood clot or ruptured blood vessel. It is vital that the casualty is taken to hospital quickly. If the stroke is due to a clot, drugs can be given to limit the extent of the damage to the brain tissue and promote recovery.

Strokes are more common in later life and in people with circulatory disorders. The effect of a stroke depends on the extent of the damage to the brain. The condition can be fatal in some cases; however, many people make a complete recovery.

RECOGNITION

There may be:
- Problems with speech and swallowing.
- If asked to show teeth, only one side of mouth will move or movement will be uneven.
- Loss of power or movement in the limbs.
- Sudden, severe headache.
- Confused, emotional mental state that could be mistaken for drunkenness.
- Sudden or gradual loss of consciousness.

▶ See also LIFE-SAVING PROCEDURES pp.19–48

✚ YOUR AIMS

- To maintain an open airway.
- To arrange urgent removal of the casualty to hospital.

❶ WARNING

If the casualty is unconscious, open the airway and check breathing; be prepared to give rescue breaths and start chest compressions if needed (see LIFE-SAVING PROCEDURES, pp.19–48).

If she is breathing, place her in the recovery position (pp.30–31).

DIAL 999 FOR AN AMBULANCE

Monitor and record vital signs – level of response, pulse, and breathing (pp.8–9) – until medical help arrives.

❶ CAUTION

Do not give the casualty anything to eat or drink because a stroke may make it difficult to swallow.

1 If the casualty is conscious, help her to lie down with her head and shoulders slightly raised and supported. Incline her head to the affected side, and place a towel on her shoulder to absorb any dribbling.
DIAL 999 FOR AN AMBULANCE

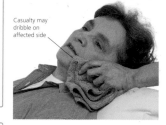

Casualty may dribble on affected side

2 Loosen any clothing that might impair the casualty's breathing. Continue to reassure her. Monitor and record vital signs – level of response, pulse, and breathing (pp.8–9) – until medical help arrives.

DIABETES MELLITUS

In this condition, the body fails to produce enough insulin, a chemical that regulates blood sugar (glucose) levels. As a result, sugar builds up in the blood, causing hyperglycaemia (below). Too much insulin or too little sugar can cause hypoglycaemia (opposite). The chart below compares both conditions. If a known diabetic casualty appears unwell, give sugar. This will correct hypoglycaemia and will do little harm in hyperglycaemia.

COMPARING HYPERGLYCAEMIA AND HYPOGLYCAEMIA

Category		Hyperglycaemia	Hypoglycaemia
History	Recent eating habits	Eaten excessively	Undereaten or missed meals
	Amount of insulin used	Not enough for amount of food eaten	Too much for amount of food eaten
	Speed of onset of symptoms	Gradual	Rapid
Symptoms	Thirst	Present	Absent
	Hunger	Absent	Present
	Vomiting	Common	Uncommon
	Urination	Excessive	Normal
Signs	Odour on the breath	Fruity/sweet	Normal
	Breathing	Rapid	Normal
	Pulse	Rapid and weak	Rapid and strong
	Skin	Warm and dry	Pale and cold, with sweating
	Seizures	Uncommon	Common
	Level of consciousness	Drowsy	Rapid loss of consciousness

HYPERGLYCAEMIA

High blood sugar (hyperglycaemia) over a long period can result in unconsciousness. In most cases, the casualty will drift into this state over a few days. Hyperglycaemia requires urgent treatment in hospital.

RECOGNITION

- Warm, dry skin; rapid pulse and breathing.
- Fruity/sweet breath and excessive thirst.
- If untreated, drowsiness, then unconsciousness.

+ YOUR AIM

- To arrange urgent removal of the casualty to hospital.

1 **DIAL 999 FOR AN AMBULANCE**
If the casualty is unconscious, place him in the recovery position (pp.30–31).

2 Monitor and record vital signs – level of response, pulse, and breathing (pp.8–9).

HYPOGLYCAEMIA

When the blood-sugar level falls below normal (hypoglycaemia), brain function is affected. This problem is characterised by a rapidly deteriorating level of response. Hypoglycaemia can occur in people with diabetes mellitus and, more rarely, appear with an epileptic seizure or after an episode of binge drinking. It can also complicate heat exhaustion or hypothermia.

People with diabetes mellitus may carry their own blood-testing kits with which to check their blood-sugar levels, and many diabetics carry sugar lumps or a tube of glucose in gel form in case they feel they are having a "hypo".

If the hypoglycaemic attack is at an advanced stage, consciousness may be impaired or lost and you must get emergency help immediately.

RECOGNITION

There may be:
- A history of diabetes; the casualty may recognise the onset of a "hypo" attack.
- Weakness, faintness, or hunger.
- Palpitations and muscle tremors.
- Strange actions or behaviour; the casualty may seem confused or belligerent.
- Sweating and cold, clammy skin.
- Pulse may be rapid and strong.
- Deteriorating level of response.
- Diabetic's warning card, glucose gel, tablets, or an insulin syringe among casualty's possessions.

▶ See also HEAT EXHAUSTION p.105
● HYPOTHERMIA pp.108–110 ● LIFE-SAVING
PROCEDURES pp.19–48 ● SEIZURES IN
ADULTS pp.94–95

✚ YOUR AIMS

- To raise the sugar content of the blood as quickly as possible.
- To obtain medical aid if necessary.

❗ WARNING

- If consciousness is impaired, do not give the casualty anything to eat or drink.
- If the casualty is unconscious, open the airway and check breathing; be ready to give rescue breaths and chest compressions if necessary (see LIFE-SAVING PROCEDURES, pp.19–48). If she is breathing, place her in the recovery position.

DIAL 999 FOR AN AMBULANCE

Monitor and record the vital signs – level of response, pulse, and breathing (pp.8–9).

1 Help the casualty to sit or lie down. Give her a sugary drink, sugar lumps, chocolate, or other sweet food; or, if she has her own glucose gel, help her to take it.

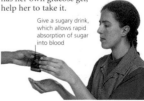

Give a sugary drink, which allows rapid absorption of sugar into blood

2 If the casualty responds quickly, give more food or drink, and let her rest until she feels better. Advise her to see her doctor even if she feels fully recovered. If her condition does not improve, you should monitor her level of response (p.8) and look for other possible causes.

SEIZURES IN ADULTS

When many muscles in the body contract involuntarily, this is known as a seizure, a convulsion, or a fit. The condition is due to a disturbance in the electrical activity of the brain. Seizures usually result in loss or impairment of consciousness. The most common cause is epilepsy. Other causes include head injury, some brain-damaging diseases, shortage of oxygen or glucose in the brain, and intake of certain poisons, including alcohol.

Epileptic seizures are due to recurrent, major disturbances of brain activity. Just before a seizure, a casualty may have a brief warning period (aura) with, for example, a strange feeling or a smell or taste.

Care must include maintaining an open, clear airway and monitoring the casualty's vital signs – level of response, pulse, and breathing. You will also need to protect the casualty from further harm during a seizure and arrange aftercare once he has recovered.

RECOGNITION

Generally:
- Sudden unconsciousness.
- Rigidity and arching of the back.
- Convulsive movements.

In epilepsy the sequence below is common:
- The casualty suddenly falls unconscious, often letting out a cry.
- He becomes rigid, arching his back.
- Breathing may cease. The lips may show a grey–blue tinge (cyanosis) and the face and neck may become red and puffy.
- Convulsive movements begin. The jaw may be clenched, breathing may be noisy, and saliva – bloodstained if the mouth has been bitten – may appear. There may be loss of bladder or bowel control.
- Muscles relax, breathing becomes normal; the casualty recovers consciousness, usually within minutes. He may feel dazed, act strangely, and be unaware of his actions.
- After a seizure, the casualty may feel tired and fall into a deep sleep.

▶ See also LIFE-SAVING PROCEDURES pp.19–48

➕ YOUR AIMS

- To protect the casualty from injury.
- To give care when consciousness is regained.
- To get casualty to hospital if necessary.

1 If you see the casualty falling, try to ease her fall. Make space around her and ask bystanders to move away. Remove potentially dangerous items, such as hot drinks and sharp objects. Note the time when the seizure started.

2 If possible, protect the casualty's head by placing soft padding underneath it. Loosen clothing around her neck.

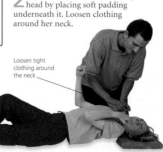

Loosen tight clothing around the neck

3 When the seizure has ceased, open the airway and check breathing; be ready to give rescue breaths and chest compressions if necessary (*see* LIFE-SAVING PROCEDURES, pp.19–48).

4 If she is breathing, place her in the recovery position. Monitor and record vital signs – level of response, pulse, and breathing (pp.8–9). Note the duration of the seizure.

❶ CAUTION

• Do not move the casualty unless she is in immediate danger.

• Do not put anything in her mouth or use force to restrain her.

❶ WARNING

If any of the following apply

DIAL 999 FOR AN AMBULANCE

• The casualty is unconscious for more than 10 minutes.

• The seizure continues for more than 5 minutes.

• The casualty is having repeated seizures or having her first seizure.

• The casualty is not aware of any reason for the seizure.

ABSENCE SEIZURES

Some people experience a mild form of epilepsy: seizures during which they seem unaware of their surroundings. These "absence seizures" tend to affect children more than adults. Convulsions or loss of consciousness are unlikely, but a full seizure may follow.

RECOGNITION

• Sudden "switching off"; the casualty may stare blankly ahead.

• Slight or localised twitching or jerking of the lips, eyelids, head, or limbs.

• Odd "automatic" movements, such as lip-smacking, chewing, or making noises.

➕ YOUR AIM

• To protect the casualty from harm until she is fully recovered.

1 Help the casualty to sit down in a quiet place. Make space around her; remove any potentially dangerous items, such as hot drinks and sharp objects.

2 Talk to the casualty in a calm and reassuring way. Stay with her until you are sure that she is fully recovered.

3 If the casualty does not recognise or have any awareness of her condition, advise her to consult her own doctor as soon as possible.

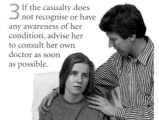

SEIZURES IN CHILDREN

In young children, seizures – also called fits or convulsions – are often the result of a raised body temperature associated with a throat or ear infection or other infectious disease. This type of seizure is known as a febrile convulsion and is a reaction of the brain to high body temperature. Epilepsy is another possible cause of seizures in infants and children.

Seizures can be alarming but they are rarely dangerous. However, the child should be seen at a hospital to rule out any serious underlying condition.

See also UNCONSCIOUS CHILD pp.32–39

RECOGNITION

- Violent muscle twitching, with clenched fists and an arched back.
There may also be:
- Obvious signs of fever: hot, flushed skin, and perhaps sweating.
- Twitching of the face with squinting, fixed, or upturned eyes.
- Breath-holding, with red, "puffy" face and neck or drooling at the mouth.
- Loss or impairment of consciousness.

+ YOUR AIMS

- To protect the child from injury.
- To cool the child.
- To reassure the parents or carer.
- To arrange removal to hospital.

1 Position pillows or soft padding around the child so that even violent movement will not result in injury.

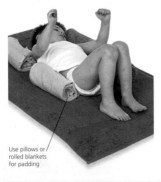

Use pillows or rolled blankets for padding

2 Remove any covering or clothes. Ensure a good supply of cool, fresh air (but do not over-cool the child).

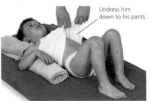

Undress him down to his pants

3 Sponge the child's skin with tepid water to help cooling; start at his forehead and work down his body.

4 Once the seizures have stopped, keep the airway open by placing the child in the recovery position (pp.38–39) if necessary.
DIAL 999 FOR AN AMBULANCE

5 Reassure the child and parents or carer. Monitor and record vital signs – level of response, pulse, and breathing (pp.8–9) – until medical help arrives.

7

THIS CHAPTER DEALS with the effects of injuries and illnesses caused by environmental factors such as extremes of heat and cold.

The skin protects the body and helps to maintain body temperature within a normal range. It can be damaged by fire, hot liquids, or caustic substances. Such injuries are often sustained in incidents such as explosions or chemical spillages.

The effects of temperature extremes can also impair skin and other body functions. The injuries may be localised – as in frostbite or sunburn – or generalised, as in heat exhaustion or hypothermia.

CONTENTS

Severe burns and scalds 98

Minor burns and scalds 100

Burns to the airway 101

Electrical burn 102

Chemical burn 103

Chemical burn to the eye 104

Heat exhaustion 105

Heatstroke 106

Frostbite 107

Hypothermia 108

ENVIRONMENTAL INJURIES

✚ FIRST-AID PRIORITIES

- Assess the casualty's condition.
- Comfort and reassure the casualty.
- Obtain medical aid if necessary. Call an ambulance if you suspect a serious illness or injury.

BURNS
- Protect yourself and the casualty from danger.
- Assess the burn, prevent further damage, and relieve symptoms.

EXTREME TEMPERATURES
- Protect the casualty from heat or cold.
- Restore normal body temperature.

SEVERE BURNS AND SCALDS

Take great care when treating burns that are deep or extensive. If the casualty has been burnt in a fire, assume that smoke or hot air has also affected the respiratory system (*see* BURNS TO THE AIRWAY, p.101).

The priorities are to begin rapid cooling of the burn and to check breathing. A casualty with a severe burn or scald is likely to be suffering from shock and will need hospital care.

The possibility of non-accidental injury must always be considered, no matter what the age of the casualty.

▶ See also BURNS TO THE AIRWAY p.101
● LIFE-SAVING PROCEDURES pp.19–48
● SHOCK pp.50–51

RECOGNITION

There may be:
● Pain.
● Difficulty breathing.
● Signs of shock (pp.50–51).

Record all details accurately and retain any clothing that has been removed in case of future investigation.

✚ YOUR AIMS

● To stop the burning and relieve pain.
● To maintain an open airway.
● To treat associated injuries.
● To minimise the risk of infection.
● To arrange urgent removal to hospital and to gather information for the emergency services.

❶ WARNING

Watch for signs of difficulty breathing; be prepared to give rescue breaths and chest compressions if necessary (see LIFE-SAVING PROCEDURES, pp.19–48).

1 Help the casualty to lie down. Try to prevent the burnt area from coming into contact with the ground.

2 Douse the burn with plenty of cold liquid for at least 10 minutes, but do not allow this to delay the casualty's removal to hospital.
DIAL 999 FOR AN AMBULANCE

3 Continue cooling the affected area until the pain is relieved.

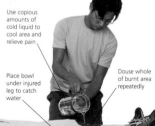

Use copious amounts of cold liquid to cool area and relieve pain

Place bowl under injured leg to catch water

Douse whole of burnt area repeatedly

4 Put on disposable gloves if available. Gently remove any rings, watches, belts, shoes, or smouldering clothing before the tissues begin to swell. Carefully remove any burnt clothing, unless it is sticking to the burn.

Remove clothing around site of burn

Use blunt-tipped scissors to cut clothing

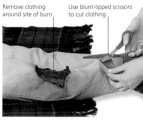

5 Cover the injured area with a sterile wound dressing to protect it from infection. If you do not have a sterile dressing, use a folded triangular bandage, part of a sheet, or kitchen film (discard the first two turns from the roll and apply it lengthways over the burn). You can use a clean plastic bag to cover a hand or foot; secure it with a bandage or adhesive tape applied over the plastic, not the skin.

SPECIAL CASE

BURNS TO THE FACE
If the casualty has a facial burn, do not cover the injury; you could cause the casualty distress and obstruct the airway. Keep cooling the area with water to relieve the pain until help arrives.

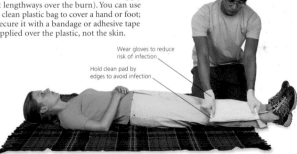

Wear gloves to reduce risk of infection

Hold clean pad by edges to avoid infection

6 Gather and record details of the casualty's injuries. Monitor and record her vital signs – level of response, pulse, and breathing (pp.8–9).

7 While waiting for help to arrive, reassure the casualty and treat her for shock (pp.50–51) if necessary.

MINOR BURNS AND SCALDS

Small, superficial burns and scalds are often due to domestic incidents, such as touching a hot iron or spilling boiling water on the skin. Most minor burns can be treated by first aid and will heal naturally. However, you should advise the casualty to see a doctor if you are at all concerned about the severity of the injury.

Some time after a burn, blisters may form. These thin "bubbles" are caused by tissue fluid (serum) leaking into the burnt area just beneath the skin's surface. Do not break a blister: you may introduce infection into the wound.

YOUR AIMS

- To stop the burning.
- To relieve pain and swelling.
- To minimise the risk of infection.

❶ CAUTION

- Do not break blisters or otherwise interfere with the injured area.
- Do not apply adhesive dressings or adhesive tape to the skin; the burn may be more extensive than it first appears.
- Do not apply ointments or fats; they may damage tissues and increase the risk of infection.

1 Flood the injured part with cold water for at least 10 minutes to stop the burning and relieve the pain. This is more effective than using sprays. If water is not available, use any cold, harmless liquid, such as milk or canned drinks.

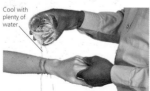

Cool with plenty of water.

2 Put on disposable gloves if available. Gently remove jewellery, watches, belts, or constricting clothing from the injured area before it begins to swell.

3 Cover the area with a sterile wound dressing or a clean, non-fluffy pad, and bandage loosely in place. A plastic bag or kitchen film makes a good temporary covering. Apply kitchen film lengthways to prevent constriction of the area if the tissues swell.

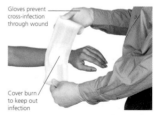

Gloves prevent cross-infection through wound

Cover burn to keep out infection

SPECIAL CASE

BLISTERS
A blister usually needs no treatment. However, if the blister breaks or may burst, apply a non-adhesive dressing that extends well beyond the edges of the blister. Leave in place until the blister subsides.

BURNS TO THE AIRWAY

Burns to the face, and within the mouth or throat, are very serious because the air passages rapidly become swollen. Signs of burning will usually be evident. However, damage to the airway must be suspected if the casualty has been burned in a confined space because he is likely to have inhaled hot air or gases.

For an extreme case, there is no specific first-aid treatment; swelling will rapidly block the airway, and there is a serious risk of suffocation. Immediate medical aid is required.

RECOGNITION

There may be:
● Soot around the nose or mouth.
● Singeing of the nasal hairs.
● Redness, swelling, or actual burning of the tongue.
● Damage to the skin around the mouth.
● Hoarseness of the voice.
● Breathing difficulties.

▶ See also LIFE-SAVING PROCEDURES pp.19–48 ● SHOCK pp.50–51

✚ YOUR AIMS

● To maintain an open airway.
● To arrange urgent removal to hospital.

❶ WARNING

If the casualty becomes unconscious, open the airway and check breathing; be prepared to give rescue breaths and chest compressions if necessary (*see* LIFE-SAVING PROCEDURES, pp.19–48). If the casualty is breathing, place him in the recovery position (pp.30–31).

1 DIAL 999 FOR AN AMBULANCE Tell the control officer that you suspect burns to the airway.

2 Take any steps possible to improve the casualty's air supply, such as loosening clothing around his neck.

3 Offer ice or small sips of cold water to reduce swelling and/or pain.

4 Reassure the casualty. Monitor and record his vital signs – level of response, pulse, and breathing (pp.8–9) – until help arrives.

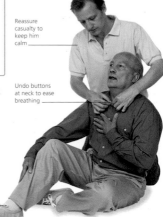

Reassure casualty to keep him calm

Undo buttons at neck to ease breathing

ELECTRICAL BURN

Burns may occur when electricity passes through the body. While visible damage occurs at the points of entry and exit of the current, there may also be internal damage. The position and direction of entry and exit wounds will alert you to the likely site and extent of hidden injury and to the degree of shock the casualty may suffer.

An electric shock can also cause cardiac arrest. If the casualty is unconscious, your immediate priority, once you are sure the area is safe, is to open the casualty's airway and check for breathing and circulation.

RECOGNITION

There may be:
- Unconsciousness.
- Full-thickness burns, with swelling, scorching, and charring, at the points of entry and exit.
- Signs of shock.
- A brown, coppery residue on the skin if the casualty has been a victim of "arcing" high-voltage electricity. (Do not mistake this residue for injury.)

▶ See also LIFE-SAVING PROCEDURES pp.19–48 ● SEVERE BURNS AND SCALDS pp.98–99 ● SHOCK pp.50–51

➕ YOUR AIMS

- To treat the burns and shock.
- To arrange urgent removal to hospital.

1 Before touching the casualty, first make sure that contact with the electrical source is broken.

2 Flood the sites of injury, at the entry and exit points of the current, with plenty of cold water to cool the burns.

3 Put on disposable gloves if available. Place a sterile wound dressing, a clean, folded triangular bandage, or clean, non-fluffy material over the burns to protect them against airborne infection. **DIAL 999 FOR AN AMBULANCE**

4 Reassure the casualty and treat him for shock (pp.50–51).

❶ CAUTION

Do not approach a victim of high-voltage electricity unless you are officially informed that the current is switched off and isolated.

❶ WARNING

If the casualty is unconscious, open the airway and check breathing; be prepared to give rescue breaths and chest compressions if necessary (see LIFE-SAVING PROCEDURES, pp.19–48).

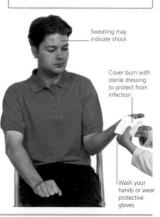

Sweating may indicate shock

Cover burn with sterile dressing to protect from infection

Wash your hands or wear protective gloves

CHEMICAL BURN

Certain chemicals may irritate, burn, or penetrate the skin, causing widespread and sometimes fatal damage. Unlike burns caused by heat, signs of chemical burns develop slowly, but the first aid is similar.

Most strong, corrosive chemicals are found in industry, but chemical burns can also occur in the home, especially from dishwasher products, oven cleaners, and paint stripper. Such burns are always serious and may require urgent hospital treatment. If possible, note the name or brand of the burning substance. Always safeguard your own and others' health: some chemicals give off poisonous fumes.

RECOGNITION

There may be:
- Evidence of chemicals in the vicinity.
- Intense, stinging pain.
- Later, discoloration, blistering, peeling, and swelling of the affected area.

✚ YOUR AIMS

- To make the area safe and inform the relevant authority.
- To disperse the harmful chemical.
- To arrange transport to hospital.

❶ CAUTION

- Never attempt to neutralise acid or alkali burns unless trained to do so.
- Do not delay starting treatment by searching for an antidote.

4 Arrange to take or send the casualty to hospital. Make sure that the airway is open. Monitor vital signs – level of response, pulse, and breathing (pp.8–9). Pass on details of the chemical to medical staff. If in the workplace, notify the safety officer and/or emergency services.

1 Make sure that the area around the casualty is safe. Ventilate the area to disperse fumes, and, if possible, seal the chemical container. Remove the casualty if necessary.

2 Flood the burn with water for at least 20 minutes to disperse the chemical and stop the burning. If treating a casualty on the ground, ensure that the water does not collect underneath her.

3 Gently remove any contaminated clothing while flooding the injury.

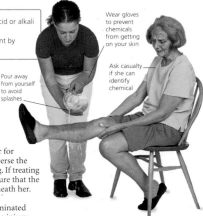

Pour away from yourself to avoid splashes

Wear gloves to prevent chemicals from getting on your skin

Ask casualty if she can identify chemical

CHEMICAL BURN TO THE EYE

Splashes of chemicals in the eye can cause serious injury if not treated quickly. They can damage the surface of the eye, resulting in scarring and even blindness.

The priority is to wash out (irrigate) the eye so that the chemical is diluted and dispersed. When irrigating the eye, put on protective gloves, if available, and avoid splashing contaminated rinsing water on you or the casualty.

RECOGNITION

There may be:
- Intense pain in the eye.
- Inability to open the injured eye.
- Redness and swelling around the eye.
- Copious watering of the eye.
- Evidence of chemical substances or containers in the immediate area.

+ YOUR AIMS

- To disperse the harmful chemical.
- To arrange transport to hospital.

❶ CAUTION

Do not allow the casualty to touch the injured eye or remove a contact lens.

1 Put on protective gloves if available. Hold the casualty's affected eye under gently running cold water for at least 10 minutes. Take care to irrigate the eyelid thoroughly both inside and out. You may find it easier to pour the water over the eye using an eye irrigator or a glass.

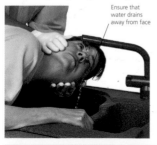

Ensure that water drains away from face

2 If the eye is shut in a spasm of pain, gently but firmly pull the eyelids open. Be very careful that contaminated water does not splash the uninjured eye.

3 Ask the casualty to hold a sterile eye dressing or a clean, non-fluffy pad over the injured eye. If it will be some time before the casualty receives medical attention, bandage the pad loosely in position.

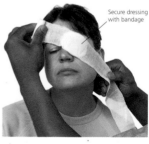

Secure dressing with bandage

4 Identify the chemical if possible. Then arrange to take or send the casualty to hospital.

HEAT EXHAUSTION

This disorder is caused by loss of salt and water from the body through excessive sweating. Heat exhaustion usually affects people who are not acclimatised to hot, humid conditions; people who are ill with vomiting or diarrhoea are particularly susceptible.

A dangerous and common cause of heat exhaustion is the excessively high body temperature, and other physical changes, that result from taking drugs such as Ecstasy. In some cases, heat exhaustion can lead to heatstroke and may even cause death.

RECOGNITION

As the condition develops, there may be:
- Headache, dizziness, and confusion.
- Loss of appetite and nausea.
- Sweating, with pale, clammy skin.
- Cramps in the arms, legs, or the abdominal wall.
- Rapid, weakening pulse and breathing.

▶ See also HEATSTROKE p.106
● LIFE-SAVING PROCEDURES pp.19–48

YOUR AIMS
- To replace lost body fluids and salt.
- To cool the casualty down if necessary.
- To obtain medical aid if necessary.

1 Help the casualty to a cool place. Get him to lie down with raised legs.

2 Give him plenty of water; follow, if possible, with a weak salt solution (one teaspoon of salt per litre of water).

3 Even if the casualty recovers quickly, ensure that he sees a doctor. If the casualty's responses deteriorate, place him in the recovery position (pp.30–31). DIAL 999 FOR AN AMBULANCE

4 Monitor and record vital signs – level of response, pulse, and breathing (pp.8–9). Be prepared to give rescue breaths and chest compressions if necessary (see LIFE-SAVING PROCEDURES, pp.19–48).

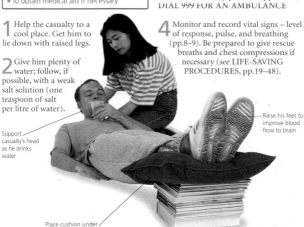

Support casualty's head as he drinks water

Place cushion under his feet for comfort

Raise his feet to improve blood flow to brain

HEATSTROKE

This condition is caused by a failure of the "thermostat" in the brain, which regulates body temperature. The body becomes seriously overheated, often due to high fever or exposure to heat. Heatstroke can also result from use of drugs such as Ecstasy. In some cases, heatstroke follows heat exhaustion when sweating ceases, and the body cannot be cooled by sweat evaporation.

Heatstroke can develop with little warning, causing unconsciousness within minutes of feeling unwell.

| RECOGNITION |

There may be:
- Headache, dizziness, and discomfort.
- Restlessness and confusion.
- Hot, flushed, and dry skin.
- Rapid deterioration in the level of response.
- Full, bounding pulse.
- Body temperature above 40°C (104°F).

▶ See also CHECKING TEMPERATURE p.9 ● DRUG POISONING p.119 ● LIFE-SAVING PROCEDURES pp.19–48

| ➕ YOUR AIMS |

- To lower the casualty's body temperature as quickly as possible.
- To arrange urgent removal to hospital.

1 Quickly move the casualty to a cool place. Remove as much of his outer clothing as possible.
DIAL 999 FOR AN AMBULANCE

2 Wrap the casualty in a cold, wet sheet and keep the sheet wet until his temperature falls to 38°C (100.4°F) under the tongue, or 37.5°C (99.5°F) under the armpit. If no sheet is available, fan the casualty, or sponge him with cold water.

3 Once the casualty's temperature appears to have returned to normal, replace the wet sheet with a dry one.

4 Monitor and record vital signs – level of response, pulse, and breathing (pp.8–9) – until help arrives. If his temperature rises again, repeat the cooling process.

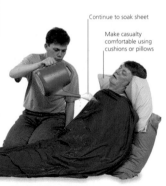

Continue to soak sheet

Make casualty comfortable using cushions or pillows

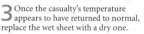

| ⚠ WARNING |

If the casualty becomes unconscious, open the airway and check breathing; be prepared to give rescue breaths and chest compressions if necessary (see LIFE-SAVING PROCEDURES, pp.19–48). If the casualty is breathing, place him in the recovery position (pp.30–31).

FROSTBITE

With this condition, the tissues of the extremities – usually the fingers and toes – freeze due to low temperatures. In severe cases, this freezing can lead to permanent loss of sensation and gangrene (tissue death) as the blood vessels become permanently damaged.

Frostbite usually occurs in freezing or cold and windy conditions. People who are unable to move around are particularly susceptible. In many cases, frostbite is accompanied by hypothermia (pp.108–110).

See also HYPOTHERMIA pp.108–110

RECOGNITION

There may be:
- At first, "pins-and-needles".
- Pallor, followed by numbness.
- Hardening and stiffening of the skin.
- A colour change to the skin of the affected area: first white, then mottled and blue. On recovery, the skin may be red, hot, painful, and blistered. Where gangrene occurs, the tissue may become black due to loss of blood supply.

YOUR AIMS

- To warm the affected area slowly to prevent further tissue damage.
- To arrange transport to hospital.

1 If possible, move the casualty into warmth before you thaw the affected part. Do not place the part close to a source of direct heat.

2 Gently remove gloves, rings, and any other constrictions, such as boots. Warm the affected part with your hands, in your lap, or in the casualty's armpits. Avoid rubbing the affected area because this can damage skin and other tissues.

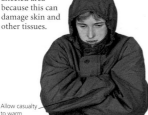

Allow casualty to warm affected part

3 Place the affected part in warm water at around 40°C (104°F). Dry carefully, and apply a light dressing of fluffed-up, dry gauze bandage.

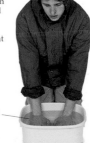

Use water that is warm but not hot

4 Raise and support the affected limb to reduce swelling. An adult may take two paracetamol tablets for intense pain. Take or send the casualty to hospital.

CAUTION

- Do not put the affected part near to a source of direct heat.
- Do not attempt to thaw the affected part if there is danger of it refreezing.
- Do not allow the casualty to smoke.

HYPOTHERMIA

This develops when the body temperature falls below 35°C (95°F). The effects vary depending on the speed of onset and the level to which the body temperature falls. Moderate hypothermia can usually be reversed. Severe hypothermia – when the core body temperature falls below 30°C (86°F) – can be fatal.

RECOGNITION

As hypothermia develops there may be:
- Shivering, and cold, pale, dry skin.
- Apathy, disorientation, or irrational behaviour; occasionally, belligerence.
- Lethargy or impaired consciousness.
- Slow and shallow breathing.
- Slow and weakening pulse. In extreme cases, the heart may stop.

WHAT CAUSES HYPOTHERMIA
Hypothermia may develop over several days in poorly heated houses. Infants, homeless people, elderly people, and those who are thin and frail are particularly vulnerable. Lack of activity, chronic illness, and fatigue all increase the risk; alcohol and drugs can exacerbate the condition.

Hypothermia can be caused by prolonged exposure to cold out of doors, particularly when there is a high "wind-chill factor". Death from immersion in cold water may also be caused by hypothermia, not drowning.

▶ See also DROWNING p.57 ● LIFE-SAVING PROCEDURES pp.19–48

TREATMENT WHEN INDOORS

✚ YOUR AIMS

- To prevent the casualty losing any more body heat.
- To rewarm the casualty slowly.
- To obtain medical aid if necessary.

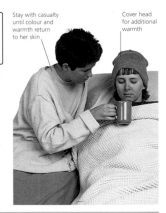

Stay with casualty until colour and warmth return to her skin

Cover head for additional warmth

1 For a casualty who has been brought in from outside, quickly replace any wet clothing with warm, dry garments.

2 The casualty can be rewarmed by bathing if she is young, fit, and able to climb into the bath unaided. The water should be warm but not too hot – about 40°C (104°F).

3 Put the casualty to bed and cover her well. Give her warm drinks, soup, or high-energy foods such as chocolate to help rewarm her.

SPECIAL CASE

HYPOTHERMIA IN THE ELDERLY

An elderly person may develop hypothermia slowly over a number of days. Elderly people often have inadequate food or heating and are more likely to suffer from chronic illness that impairs their mobility.

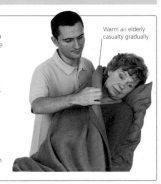

Warm an elderly casualty gradually

When treating an elderly person with hypothermia, be careful to warm her slowly. Cover her with layers of blankets in a room at about 25°C (77°F). If the casualty is warmed too rapidly, blood may be diverted suddenly from the heart and brain to the body surfaces.

Always call a doctor because hypothermia can sometimes disguise the symptoms of, or accompany, a stroke, a heart attack, or an underactive thyroid gland (hypothyroidism).

❶ CAUTION

● Do not allow an elderly casualty to have a bath to warm her up – the sudden warming may cause blood to divert suddenly from the heart and brain to the body surfaces.

● Do not place any heat sources, such as hot water bottles or fires, next to the casualty because these may also mobilise blood too rapidly. In addition, they may burn the casualty.

● Do not give the casualty alcohol because this will worsen the hypothermia.

● Handle the casualty gently because, in severe cases, rushed treatment or movement may cause the heart to stop.

SPECIAL CASE

HYPOTHERMIA IN INFANTS

A baby's mechanisms for regulating body temperature are under-developed, so she may develop hypothermia in a cold room. The baby's skin may look healthy but feel cold, and she may be limp, unusually quiet, and refuse to feed. Rewarm a cold baby gradually, by wrapping her in blankets and warming the room. You should always call a doctor if you suspect a baby has hypothermia.

Cover head with a hat to prevent heat from being lost

Wrap the baby in a blanket

4 Regularly monitor and record the casualty's vital signs – level of response, pulse, breathing, and temperature (pp.8–9).

5 Call a doctor if you have any doubts about the casualty's condition. If hypothermia occurs in an elderly person or a baby, you must always obtain medical aid for the casualty.

Continued on next page

HYPOTHERMIA (continued)

TREATMENT WHEN OUTDOORS

+ YOUR AIMS

- To prevent the casualty from losing more body heat.
- To rewarm the casualty.
- To obtain help.

❶ CAUTION

Do not give the casualty any alcohol to drink. This is because alcohol dilates superficial blood vessels and allows heat to escape, making hypothermia worse.

1 Take the casualty to a sheltered place as quickly as possible.

2 Remove wet clothing. Shield the casualty from the wind. Insulate him with extra clothing or blankets and cover his head. Do not give him your clothes.

❶ WARNING

If the casualty becomes unconscious, open the airway and check breathing; be prepared to give rescue breaths and chest compressions if necessary (see LIFE-SAVING PROCEDURES, pp.19–48).

3 Protect the casualty from the ground and the elements. Put him in a dry sleeping bag, cover him with blankets or newspapers and enclose him in a plastic or foil survival bag, if available.

Lay casualty on a thick layer of dry insulating material, such as pine branches, heather, or bracken

Protect him from wind and rain with survival bag

Shelter and warm him with your body

4 Send for help. In an ideal situation, two people should go together for help. However, it is important that you do not leave the casualty alone; someone must remain with him at all times.

5 To help rewarm a casualty who is conscious, give him warm drinks, and feed him with high-energy foods such as chocolate, if you have such drinks or foods available.

6 When help arrives, the casualty should be taken to hospital by stretcher immediately.

SPECIAL CASE

WHEN NO HELP IS AVAILABLE
If you are alone with the casualty, try to attract attention by using a whistle, flashing a torch, or lighting a fire.

8

CONTENTS

Splinter 112

Embedded fish-hook..............113

Foreign object in the eye........114

Foreign object in the ear........115

Foreign object in the nose......115

Inhaled foreign object............116

Swallowed foreign object.......116

OBJECTS THAT FIND their way into the body, either through a wound in the skin or via an orifice (such as the ear, nose, or eye), are known as "foreign objects". Such items range from specks of dirt or grit in the eye to small objects that young children may push into their noses and ears. Foreign objects do not usually cause serious problems, but they can be painful and distressing. Calm, reassuring treatment is essential.

TREATMENT PROCEDURES
This chapter gives advice on how to remove objects from the skin and orifices, including what to do when something has been swallowed or inhaled. First aid for a person with an object embedded in a wound is given in Chapter 4, Wounds and Bleeding (pp.59–68).

+ FIRST-AID PRIORITIES

- Assess the casualty's condition.
- Comfort and reassure the casualty.
- Establish whether or not a foreign object can be removed safely.
- Prevent further damage.
- Obtain medical aid if necessary. Call an ambulance if you suspect a serious illness or injury.

SPLINTER

Small splinters of wood, metal, or glass may enter the top layer of skin. They carry a risk of infection because they are rarely clean. Usually, a splinter can be withdrawn from the skin using sterile tweezers. However, if the splinter is deeply embedded in the skin, lies over a joint, or is difficult to remove, you should leave it in place and advise the casualty to consult a doctor.

▶ See also FOREIGN OBJECT IN A CUT p.63

YOUR AIMS

- To remove the splinter.
- To minimise the risk of infection.

1 Sterilise a pair of tweezers by holding them in a flame and then letting them cool. Put on disposable gloves if available. Gently clean around the splinter with soap and warm water.

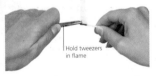

Hold tweezers in flame

2 Grasp the splinter with the tweezers as close to the skin as possible, and draw it out at the angle at which it went in.

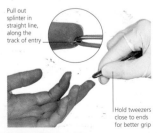

Pull out splinter in straight line, along the track of entry

Hold tweezers close to ends for better grip

SPECIAL CASE

EMBEDDED SPLINTER
If a splinter is embedded or difficult to dislodge, do not probe the area with a sharp object such as a needle or you may introduce infection. Pad around the splinter until you can bandage over it without pressing down, and seek medical advice.

3 Carefully squeeze the wound to encourage a little bleeding. This will help to flush out any remaining dirt.

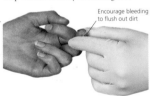

Encourage bleeding to flush out dirt

4 Clean the area, pat it dry, and apply an adhesive dressing (plaster) to minimise the risk of infection.

ⓘ CAUTION

Always ask about tetanus immunisation.
Seek medical advice if:
- The casualty has never been immunised.
- The casualty is uncertain about the timing and number of injections that have been given.
- It is more than 10 years since the casualty's last injection.

EMBEDDED FISH-HOOK

A fish-hook is barbed, which means that once embedded in the skin it is difficult to remove. Only remove a hook yourself if medical aid is not available. Embedded fish-hooks carry a risk of infection, including tetanus.

WHEN MEDICAL AID IS NOT READILY AVAILABLE

✚ YOUR AIMS
• To remove the fish-hook without causing the casualty any further injury and pain.

❶ WARNING
Do not try to pull out a fish-hook unless you can cut off the barb. If you cannot, seek medical help.

1 Put on disposable gloves if available. If the barb is visible, use wire cutters to cut it away; carefully withdraw the hook by its eye.

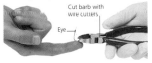

Cut barb with wire cutters

Eye

2 Clean the wound, then pad around it with gauze and bandage it.

SPECIAL CASE
BARB NOT VISIBLE
Push the hook further in until the barb emerges. Cut off the barb, and remove the hook (left). If you cannot do this, seek medical help.

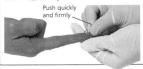

Push quickly and firmly

❶ CAUTION
Always ask about tetanus immunisation.
Seek medical advice if:
• The casualty has never been immunised.
• The casualty is uncertain about the timing and number of injections that have been given.
• It is more than 10 years since the casualty's last injection.

WHEN MEDICAL AID IS READILY AVAILABLE

✚ YOUR AIMS
• To obtain medical aid.
• To minimise the risk of infection.

1 Put on disposable gloves if available. Ask the casualty to sit down and support the injured area. Cut off the fishing line, being careful to make the cut as close to the hook as possible.

2 Build up pads of gauze around the hook until you can bandage over it without pushing it in further.

Ensure top of padding is level with top of hook

3 Bandage over the padding and the hook; take care not to press down on the hook. See that the casualty receives medical attention as soon as possible.

FOREIGN OBJECT IN THE EYE

A speck of dust, a loose eyelash, or even a contact lens can float on the white of the eye. Usually, such objects can easily be rinsed off. However, you must not touch anything that sticks to the eye, penetrates the eyeball, or rests on the coloured part of the eye (iris and pupil) because this may damage the eye. Instead, make sure that the casualty gets medical attention quickly.

RECOGNITION

There may be:
- Blurred vision.
- Pain or discomfort.
- Redness and watering of the eye.
- Eyelids screwed up in spasm.

See also EYE WOUND p.65

+ YOUR AIM

- To prevent injury to the eye.

❶ CAUTION

Do not touch anything that is sticking to, or embedded in, the eyeball or over the coloured part of the eye. Cover the eye (*see* EYE WOUND, p.65) and take or send the casualty to hospital.

1 Advise the casualty to sit down facing the light; tell her not to rub her eye. Stand behind the casualty.

2 Gently separate her eyelids with your finger and thumb. Examine every part of her eye carefully.

3 If you can see a foreign object on the white of the eye, wash it out by pouring clean water from a glass or by using a sterile eyewash.

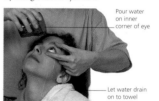

Pour water on inner corner of eye

Let water drain on to towel

4 If this is unsuccessful, lift the object off with a moist swab or the damp corner of a tissue. If you still cannot remove the object, seek medical help.

SPECIAL CASE

OBJECT UNDER UPPER EYELID
Ask the casualty to grasp her lashes and pull the upper lid over the lower lid. Blinking under water may also make the object float off.

Lower lashes may brush particle clear

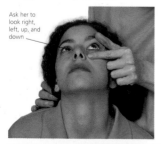

Ask her to look right, left, up, and down

FOREIGN OBJECT IN THE EAR

If a foreign object becomes lodged in the ear, it may block the ear canal and cause temporary deafness. In some cases, a foreign object may damage the eardrum. Young children frequently push objects into their ears. Insects can also fly or crawl into the ear and may cause alarm.

✚ YOUR AIMS

- To prevent injury to the ear.
- To remove a trapped insect if it is moving.
- To arrange transport to hospital if a foreign object is lodged in the ear.

1 Arrange to take or send the casualty to hospital. Do not try to remove a lodged foreign object yourself.

2 Reassure the casualty during the journey or until medical help arrives.

❶ CAUTION

Do not attempt to remove any object that is lodged in the ear. You may cause serious injury and push the object in even further.

SPECIAL CASE

INSECT INSIDE THE EAR
Reassure the casualty, and ask her to sit down. Gently flood the ear with tepid water so that the insect floats out. If this flooding does not remove the insect, take or send the casualty to hospital.

Support head, with affected ear uppermost

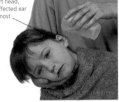

FOREIGN OBJECT IN THE NOSE

Young children may push small objects up their noses. Foreign objects can block the nose and cause infection. Sharp objects may damage the tissues, and "button" batteries can cause burns and bleeding. Do not try to remove a foreign object; you may cause injury.

RECOGNITION

There may be:
- Difficult/noisy breathing through the nose.
- Swelling of the nose.
- Smelly/blood-stained discharge, indicating that an object has been lodged for a while.

✚ YOUR AIM

- To arrange transport to hospital.

❶ CAUTION

Do not attempt to remove the foreign object, even if you can see it.

1 Keep the casualty calm. Tell him to breathe through his mouth at a normal rate. Advise him not to poke inside his nose to try to remove the object himself.

2 Arrange to take or send the casualty to hospital, where the object can safely be removed by hospital staff.

INHALED FOREIGN OBJECT

Small, smooth objects can slip past protective mechanisms in the throat and enter the air passages to the lungs. Dry peanuts, which can swell up when in contact with body fluids, pose a danger in young children; they can be inhaled into the lungs, resulting in serious damage.

People who are allergic to nuts may suffer anaphylactic shock (p.52) after swallowing them.

▶ Treat as for CHOKING ADULT p.46
● CHOKING CHILD p.47 ● CHOKING INFANT p.48

SWALLOWED FOREIGN OBJECT

Small objects such as coins, safety pins, or buttons are often swallowed by young children. They usually travel straight through the digestive tract, but there is a risk that they may enter the respiratory tract and cause choking.

Button batteries, used in some toys, watches, and hearing aids, contain corrosive chemicals; if swallowed, they can cause severe damage, and even death, if not removed. A large or sharp object may damage the digestive tract.

➕ YOUR AIM

- To obtain medical aid if necessary.

1 Reassure the casualty and try to find out exactly what she has swallowed.

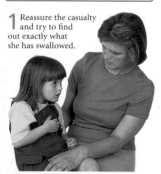

❶ WARNING

If the casualty has swallowed something large or sharp, or has difficulty breathing or swallowing
DIAL 999 FOR AN AMBULANCE
Reassure the casualty while waiting for medical help to arrive.

❶ CAUTION

Do not allow the casualty to eat, drink, or smoke because a general anaesthetic may need to be given in hospital.

2 If the swallowed object is small and smooth, arrange to take or send the casualty to hospital or to see a doctor. Always seek urgent medical advice if you know or suspect that a casualty has swallowed a battery.

9

POISONING IS USUALLY non-intentional. It may result from exposure to or ingestion of toxic substances, including drugs and alcohol, chemicals, and contaminated food. Some cases of poisoning are intentional, as in cases of attempted suicide. The effects of a poison vary depending on the type and amount of the substance absorbed. However, in most cases of poisoning, medical aid will be needed.

BITES AND STINGS

Insect stings are often minor injuries that can be treated with first aid. However, multiple insect stings can produce a very serious reaction that requires urgent medical help. Animal and human bites always need medical attention because the mouth harbours many microorganisms (germs).

CONTENTS

Swallowed poisons 118

Drug poisoning 119

Alcohol poisoning 120

Food poisoning 121

Insect sting 122

Tick bite 122

Snake bite 123

Animal bite 124

POISONING, BITES, AND STINGS

+ FIRST-AID PRIORITIES

- Assess the casualty's condition.
- Identify the poisonous substance.
- Ensure the safety of yourself and the casualty.
- Comfort and reassure the casualty.
- Obtain medical aid if necessary. Call an ambulance if you suspect a serious illness or injury.

SWALLOWED POISONS

Chemicals that are swallowed may harm the digestive tract, or cause more widespread damage if they enter the bloodstream. Hazardous chemicals include common household substances such as bleach, dishwasher detergent, and paint stripper.

Drugs, whether prescribed or bought over the counter, are also potentially harmful if they are taken in overdose. The effects of poisoning depend on the substance that has been swallowed.

▶ See also CHEMICAL BURN p.103
● DRUG POISONING p.119 ● LIFE-SAVING
PROCEDURES pp.19–48

RECOGNITION

Depends on the poison, but there may be:
● Vomiting, sometimes bloodstained.
● Impaired consciousness.
● Pain or burning sensation.
● Empty containers in the vicinity.
● History of ingestion/exposure.

YOUR AIMS

● To maintain the airway, breathing, and circulation.
● To remove any contaminated clothing.
● To identify the poison.
● To arrange urgent removal to hospital.

SPECIAL CASE

BURNED LIPS
If the casualty's lips are burned by corrosive substances, give her frequent sips of cold milk or water while waiting for medical help.

1 If the casualty is conscious, ask her what she has swallowed, and try to reassure her.

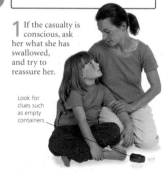

Look for clues such as empty containers

❶ WARNING

● Never attempt to induce vomiting.
● If the casualty becomes unconscious, open the airway and check breathing; be prepared to give rescue breaths and chest compressions if necessary (*see* LIFE-SAVING PROCEDURES, pp.19–48). If she is breathing, place her in the recovery position (pp.30–31).

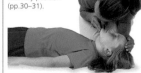

● Use a face shield or pocket mask (p.24) for rescue breathing if there are any chemicals on the casualty's mouth.

2 DIAL 999 FOR AN AMBULANCE Give as much information as possible about the swallowed poison. This information will assist doctors to give appropriate treatment once the casualty reaches hospital.

DRUG POISONING

Poisoning can result from an overdose of either prescribed drugs or drugs that are bought over the counter. It can also be caused by drug abuse or drug interaction. The effects vary depending on the type of drug and how it is taken (below). When you call the emergency services, give as much information as possible.

▶ See also LIFE-SAVING PROCEDURES pp.19–48

RECOGNITION

Category	Drug	Effects of poisoning
Painkillers	Aspirin (swallowed)	Upper abdominal pain, nausea, and vomiting ● Ringing in the ears ● "Sighing" when breathing ● Confusion and delirium ● Dizziness
	Paracetamol (swallowed)	Little effect at first, but abdominal pain, nausea, and vomiting may develop ● Irreversible liver damage may occur within 3 days (malnourishment and alcohol increase the risk)
Nervous system depressants and tranquillisers	Barbiturates and benzodiazepines (swallowed)	Lethargy and sleepiness, leading to unconsciousness ● Shallow breathing ● Weak, irregular, or abnormally slow or fast pulse
Stimulants and hallucinogens	Amphetamines (including Ecstasy) and LSD (swallowed), cocaine (inhaled)	Excitable, hyperactive behaviour, wildness, and frenzy ● Sweating ● Tremor of the hands ● Hallucinations, in which the casualty may claim to "hear voices" or "see things"
Narcotics	Morphine, heroin (commonly injected)	Small pupils ● Sluggishness and confusion, possibly leading to unconsciousness ● Slow, shallow breathing, which may stop altogether ● Needle marks, which may be infected
Solvents	Glue, lighter fuel (inhaled)	Nausea and vomiting ● Headaches ● Hallucinations ● Possibly, unconsciousness ● Rarely, cardiac arrest

✚ YOUR AIMS

● To maintain breathing and circulation.
● To arrange removal to hospital.

❶ WARNING

● If the casualty is unconscious, open the airway and check breathing; be prepared to give rescue breaths and chest compressions if necessary (see LIFE-SAVING PROCEDURES, pp.19–48). If breathing, place in the recovery position (pp.30–31).

DIAL 999 FOR AN AMBULANCE

● Do not induce vomiting.

1 If the casualty is conscious, help him into a comfortable position and ask what he has taken. Reassure him while you talk to him.

2 DIAL 999 FOR AN AMBULANCE Monitor and record vital signs – level of response, pulse, and breathing (pp.8–9) – until medical help arrives.

3 Keep samples of any vomited material. Look for evidence to help identify the drug, such as empty containers. Hand over these samples and containers to the paramedic or ambulance crew.

ALCOHOL POISONING

Prolonged or excessive intake of alcohol (chemical name, ethanol) can severely impair all physical and mental functions, and the person may sink into deep unconsciousness.

There are several risks to the casualty from alcohol poisoning:
- An unconscious casualty risks inhaling and choking on vomit.
- Alcohol widens (dilates) the blood vessels. This means that the body loses heat, and hypothermia may develop.
- A casualty who smells of alcohol may be misdiagnosed and so not be treated appropriately for an underlying cause of unconsciousness, such as a head injury, stroke, or heart attack.

▶ See also HYPOTHERMIA pp.108–110
● LIFE-SAVING PROCEDURES pp.19–48

RECOGNITION

There may be:
- A strong smell of alcohol.
- Impaired consciousness: the casualty may respond if roused, but will quickly relapse.
- Flushed and moist face.
- Deep, noisy breathing.
- Full, bounding pulse.
- Unconsciousness.

In the later stages of unconsciousness:
- Dry, bloated appearance to the face.
- Shallow breathing.
- Weak, rapid pulse.
- Dilated pupils that react poorly to light.

✛ YOUR AIMS
- To maintain an open airway.
- To assess for other conditions.
- To seek medical help if necessary.

❶ WARNING
- If the casualty is unconscious, open the airway and check breathing; be prepared to give rescue breaths and start chest compressions if necessary (see LIFE-SAVING PROCEDURES, pp.19–48). If the casualty is breathing, place him in the recovery position (pp.30–31).

DIAL 999 FOR AN AMBULANCE
- Do not induce vomiting.

1 Cover the casualty with a coat or blanket to protect him from the cold.

2 Assess the casualty for any injuries, especially head injuries, or other medical conditions.

3 Regularly monitor and record vital signs – level of response, pulse, and breathing (pp.8–9) – until the casualty recovers or can be placed in the care of a responsible person.

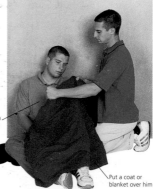

Watch casualty in case he becomes unconscious

Put a coat or blanket over him

FOOD POISONING

This is usually caused by consuming food or drink that is contaminated with bacteria or viruses. Some food poisoning is caused by poisons (toxins) from bacteria already in the food. Symptoms may develop within hours, or they may not occur until a day or so after eating contaminated food.

Toxic food poisoning is frequently caused by poisons produced by the staphylococcus group of bacteria. Symptoms usually develop rapidly, possibly within 2–6 hours of eating the affected food.

One danger of food poisoning is loss of body fluids. The dehydration

that results can be serious if fluids are not replaced quickly. Dehydration is especially serious in the very young and the very old, and, in some cases, hospital treatment may be required.

▶ See also SHOCK pp.50–51

> ✚ **YOUR AIMS**
> - To encourage the casualty to rest.
> - To give the casualty plenty of bland fluids to drink.
> - To obtain medical aid if necessary.

> ❗ **WARNING**
> If the casualty's condition worsens,
> **DIAL 999 FOR AN AMBULANCE**

1 Advise the casualty to lie down and rest. Help her if necessary.

2 Give the casualty plenty of bland fluids to drink and a bowl to use if she vomits. Call a doctor for advice.

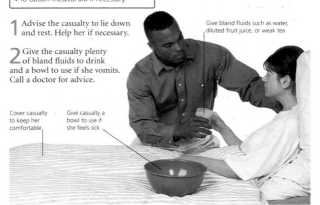

Give bland fluids such as water, diluted fruit juice, or weak tea

Cover casualty to keep her comfortable

Give casualty a bowl to use if she feels sick

INSECT STING

Usually, a sting from a bee, wasp, or hornet is painful but not dangerous. However, multiple insect stings or a sting in the mouth or throat can produce a serious reaction. With any bite or sting, watch for signs of an allergic reaction, which may lead to anaphylactic shock (p.52).

RECOGNITION

- Pain at the site of the sting.
- Redness and swelling around the site of the sting.

▶ See also ANAPHYLACTIC SHOCK p.52
● LIFE-SAVING PROCEDURES pp.19–48

✚ YOUR AIMS

- To relieve swelling and pain.
- To arrange removal to hospital if needed.

1 If the sting is visible, brush or scrape it off sideways with your fingernail or the blunt edge of a knife. Do not use tweezers; more poison may be injected into the casualty.

Brush sting off with a fingernail or blunt edge

2 Raise the affected part if possible, and apply an ice pack or cold compress (p.12) for at least 10 minutes. Advise the casualty to see her doctor if the pain and swelling persist.

❶ WARNING

If the casualty shows signs of anaphylactic shock, such as impaired breathing or swelling of the face and neck, **DIAL 999 FOR AN AMBULANCE**

SPECIAL CASE

STINGS TO THE MOUTH AND THROAT
If a casualty has been stung in the mouth, the mouth and/or throat may swell, causing blockage of the airway. To help prevent this, give the casualty an ice cube to suck or cold water to sip. If swelling develops, **DIAL 999 FOR AN AMBULANCE**

Cold water helps to reduce risk of swelling

TICK BITE

Ticks are tiny, spider-like creatures that attach themselves to passing animals (including humans) and bite into the skin to suck blood. Ticks can carry disease and cause infection, so they should be removed as soon as possible.

✚ YOUR AIM

- To remove the tick.

1 Using fine-pointed tweezers, grasp the tick's head close to the casualty's skin.

2 Use a to-and-fro action to lever the head out. Try to avoid breaking the tick and leaving the buried head behind.

3 Advise the casualty to see a doctor as soon as possible.

SNAKE BITE

The only poisonous snake native to mainland Britain is the adder, and its bite is rarely fatal. However, exotic poisonous snakes may be kept as pets. While a snake bite is not often serious, it can be frightening. The casualty should keep still to delay the spread of venom (poison) through the body. Note the snake's appearance to help doctors give the correct antivenom. Bear in mind that venom is active even if the snake is dead. If it safe to do so, put the snake in a secure container.

Depends on the species, but there may be:
- A pair of puncture marks.
- Severe pain, redness, and swelling at the site of the bite.
- Nausea, vomiting, disturbed vision.
- Increased salivation and sweating.
- Laboured breathing; in extreme cases, breathing may stop altogether.

▶ See also LIFE-SAVING PROCEDURES pp.19–48

✛ YOUR AIMS

- To prevent the spread of venom.
- To arrange urgent removal to hospital.

❶ WARNING

- Do not apply a tourniquet, slash the wound with a knife, or suck out the venom.
- If the casualty becomes unconscious, open the airway and check breathing; be prepared to give rescue breaths and chest compressions if necessary (*see* LIFE-SAVING PROCEDURES, pp.19–48).

1 Help the casualty to lie down. Reassure her, and tell her to keep calm and still. **DIAL 999 FOR AN AMBULANCE**

2 Gently wash the wound and pat dry with clean swabs.

Clean wound with gauze swab

3 Lightly compress the limb above the wound with a roller bandage. Use triangular bandages to immobilise the affected area (p.16).

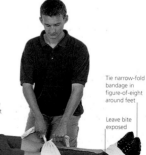

Tie narrow-fold bandage in figure-of-eight around feet

Leave bite exposed

Keep heart above the level of wounded part

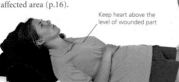

Broad-fold bandage | Soft padding | Roller bandage

123

ANIMAL BITE

Bites from sharp, pointed teeth cause deep puncture wounds that can carry bacteria and other germs far into the tissues. Any bite that breaks the skin needs prompt medical attention because of the risk of infection.

The most serious infection risk is rabies, a potentially fatal virus that is carried in the saliva of infected animals. If bitten overseas, where the risk of rabies is greatest, the casualty must receive anti-rabies injections.

Tetanus is also a potential risk following any animal bite. There is probably only a small risk of hepatitis B or C viruses being transmitted through a human bite – and an even smaller risk of transmission of the HIV (AIDS) virus. However, seek medical advice if you are concerned.

▶ See also CUTS AND GRAZES p.62
● SEVERE BLEEDING pp.60–61 ● SHOCK pp.50–51

✚ YOUR AIMS

- To control bleeding.
- To minimise the risk of infection, both to the casualty and yourself.
- To obtain medical aid if necessary.

1 Put on disposable gloves if available. Wash the bite wound thoroughly with soap and warm water in order to minimise the risk of infection.

2 Pat dry with clean gauze swabs and cover with an adhesive dressing (plaster) or a small sterile dressing.

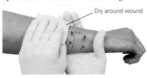

Dry around wound

3 Arrange to take or send the casualty to hospital if the wound is large or deep.

❶ WARNING

If you suspect rabies, arrange to take or send the casualty to hospital immediately.

---

❶ CAUTION

Always ask about tetanus immunisation.
Seek medical advice if:

- The casualty has never been immunised.
- The casualty is uncertain about the timing or number of injections that have been given.
- It is more than 10 years since the casualty's last injection.

SPECIAL CASE

DEEP WOUND
If the wound is deep, control bleeding by applying direct pressure and raising the injured part. Cover the wound with a non-fluffy pad, or a sterile wound dressing, and bandage in place to control bleeding. Arrange to take or send the casualty to hospital.

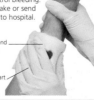

Cover wound and bandage firmly

Raise injured part

INDEX

A

abdominal wound 67
airway
  asthma 56
  burns 101
  opening of 20,
    adult 23
    child 34,
    infant 41
alcohol poisoning 120
allergic reaction and
  anaphylactic shock 52
anaphylactic shock 52
angina pectoris 53
animal bite 117, 124
ankle
  broken 86
  sprained 71, 86
arm
  injury 76
  sling 17
asthma 56

B

bandaging
  arm sling 17
  elevation sling 18
  first-aid bandages 11
  principles of 14
  reef knots 16
  roller bandages 15
  triangular bandages 16
bites 117
  animal 117, 124
  snake 123
  tick 122
bleeding 59
  abdominal 67
  cross infection, preventing 6
  cuts 62
  ear 65
  effects of loss of blood 50
  grazes 62
  head 64
  joint crease 68
  nose 66
  palm 68
  scalp 64
  severe, no object embedded
    in wound 60–61
  severe, object embedded in
    wound 61
  shock 50–51

blisters 100
body temperature, checking
  9
brain 87
  compression of 89
  concussion 88
  oxygen 19
  stroke 91
breathing, checking 9
  adult casualty 23
  child 34
  infant 42
  rescue breaths, for adult 20,
    24–25
    child 35
    infant 42–43
burns
  airway 101
  chemical 103
    to eye 104
  electrical 102
  face 99
  lips 118
  minor 100
  severe 98–99

C

cerebral compression 89
cheekbone fracture 73
chemical burn 103
  to eye 104
chest penetrating wound
  58
children
  choking 45, 47
  nosebleed 66
  seizures 96
  unconscious, resuscitation of
    32–39
choking
  adult 45, 46
  child 45, 47
  infant 45, 47
circulation, checking
  adult 26
  child 36
  infant 43
circulatory system 49
cold compresses 12
collar bone fracture 74
Colles' fracture 76
compression of the brain
  89
concussion 88

convulsions
  absence seizures 95
  adult 94–95
  children 96
  febrile 96
CPR (cardiopulmonary
  resuscitation) 20
    adult 26–27
    child 36–37
    infant 44
cross infection, preventing 6
cuts 62
  foreign object in 63

D

defibrillator 20, 28–29
diabetes mellitus 92
  hyperglycaemia 92
  hypoglycaemia 93
dislocations 71
  elbow 77
  hip 83
  shoulder 75
dressings 10
drowning 57
drug poisoning 119

E

ear
  bleeding from 65
  foreign object 115
elbow injury 77
elderly and hypothermia 109
electrical burn 102
elevation sling 18
emergency services,
  telephoning 5
emergency situation, action at
  5
environmental injuries 97–100
epilectic seizures 94
  absence seizures 95
eye
  chemical burn 104
  foreign object 114
  wounds 65
eyelid, upper
  foreign body 114

F

face burns 99
fainting 55
febrile convulsion 96
finger injuries 78

first-aid materials 10–13
  bandages 11
  cold compresses 12
  dressings 10
  home kit 11, 12
  sterile dressings 13
fish-hook, embedded 113
fits
  absence seizures 95
  adult 94–95
  child 96
fluid loss, effects of 50
food poisoning 121
foot fractures 86
foreign objects 111
  cuts 63
  ear 115
  embedded fish-hook 113
  eye 114
  eyelid 114
  inhaled 116
  nose 115
  splinter 112
  swallowed 116
fractures 70
  ankle 86
  arm 76
  cheekbone 73
  closed 70
  collar bone 74
  elbow 77
  foot 86
  hand 78
  jaw 73
  lower leg 85
  nose 73
  open 70
  pelvis 82
  skull 90
  stable 70
  thigh 83
  unstable 70
  wrist 76
frostbite 107

G

grazes 62

H

hand injuries 78
  palm wound 68
head injuries
  cerebral compression 89
  concussion 88
  skull fracture 90
  wounds 64

heart 49
  angina pectoris 53
  attack 54
  defibrillator 20, 28–29
  failure 53
heat exhaustion 105
heatstroke 106
hip injuries 83
hyperglycaemia 92
hypoglycaemia 93
hypothermia 108
  indoors, treatment 108–9
  outdoors, treatment 110

I

infants
  choking 45, 47
  hypothermia 109
  unconscious, resuscitation of
    40–44
infection, preventing cross 6
inhaled foreign object 116
injuries, types 70–71
  see also dislocations, fractures,
    wounds
insect sting 117, 122
insulin 92

J

jaw fracture 73
joint crease, wound at 68

K

knee injury 84

L

leg, lower injury 85
life-saving priorities 20
ligament injuries 71
  strains and sprains 72
lips, poison burns 118

M

monitoring vital signs 8
  breathing 9
  level of response 8
  pulse rate 8
  temperature 9
muscle injuries 71
  strains and sprains 71, 72

N

nose
  bleed 66
  foreign object 115
  fracture 73

O

overdose 119
oxygen 19

P

palm wound 68
pelvis fracture 82
penetrating chest wound 58
poisoning 117
  alcohol 120
  drug 119
  food 121
  swallowed 118
pulse rate, checking 8

R

reef knots 16
respiratory system 49
response, checking level of 8,
  adult 22
  child 33
  infant 41
resuscitation of unconscious
  adult 15, 21–31
    breathing check 23
    circulation check 26–27
    CPR 26–27
    defibrillator, use of 28–29
    opening the airway 23
    recovery position 30–31
    rescue breaths 20, 24–25
    response check 22
    sequence chart 21
resuscitation of unconscious
  child 15, 32–39
    breathing check 34
    circulation check 36
    CPR 36–7
    defibrillator, use of 28-29
    opening the airway 34
    recovery position 38–39
    rescue breaths 35
    response check 33
    sequence chart 32
resuscitation of unconscious
  infant 15, 40–44
    breathing check 42
    circulation check 43
    CPR 44
    opening the airway 41
    recovery position 44
    rescue breaths 42–43
    response check 41
    sequence chart 40
RICE procedure 72
roller bandages 15

S

scalds
 minor 100
 severe 98–99
scalp wounds 64
seizures
 absence 95
 adult 94–95
 child 96
shock 50–51
 anaphylactic 52
shoulder injury 75
skeleton 69
skull fracture 90
slings
 arm 17
 elevation 18
snake bite 123
spinal injury 79
 conscious casualty 80
 recovery position
  adult 31
  child 39
 unconscious casualty 81
splinter 112

sprains 71, 72
 ankle 86
 RICE procedure 72
sterile dressings 13
sting, insect 117, 122
strains 71, 72
 RICE procedure 72
stroke 91
swallowing
 foreign object 116
 poisons 118

T

telephoning emergency
 services 5
temperature of body,
 checking 9
tendon injuries 71
 strains and sprains 72
tetanus 62
thermometers, types 9
thigh injuries 83
tick bite 122
toe injuries 86
triangular bandages
 16

U

unconsciousness, resuscitation
 see resuscitation

W

wounds 59
 abdominal 67
 cross infection, preventing 6
 cuts 62
 cuts, foreign object in 63
 eye 65
 fish hook, embedded 113
 grazes 62
 head 64
 joint crease 68
 palm 68
 penetrating chest 58
 scalp 64
 severe bleeding, no object
  embedded in wound
  60–61
 severe bleeding, object
  embedded in wound 61
 tetanus 62
wrist fracture 76

ACKNOWLEDGMENTS

St. John Ambulance, a registered charity, St. Andrew's Ambulance Association, a registered charity in Scotland, and the British Red Cross Society, a registered charity, receive a royalty for every copy of this book sold by Dorling Kindersley. Details of the royalties payable to the Societies can be obtained by writing to the publishers, Dorling Kindersley Limited at 80 Strand, London WC2R 0RL. For the purposes of the Charities Act 1992 no further seller of the Manual shall be deemed to be a commercial participator with these three Societies.

ST. JOHN AMBULANCE

St. John Ambulance is the UK's leading first-aid, transport, and care charity. Its mission is to provide first-aid and medical support services; caring services in support of community needs; and education, training, and personal development to young people.

Call 08700 10 49 50 for details of local first-aid courses, or to find out about the many volunteering opportunities available.

ST. ANDREW'S AMBULANCE ASSOCIATION

St. Andrew's Ambulance Association is Scotland's premier provider of first-aid training and services. Every year the Association teaches over 20,000 people vital life-saving skills. Almost 2,000 volunteers give their own personal time to help others by providing first-aid cover at public events throughout Scotland. We rely heavily on donations from the public to continue our life-saving work.

BRITISH RED CROSS

The British Red Cross cares for people in crisis at home and abroad. It gives vital impartial support during both major emergencies and personal crises, and provides training in first aid and caring skills.

The red cross emblem is a symbol of protection during armed conflict and its use is restricted by law.

OBSERVATION CHARTS

Fill in the charts below when you attend a casualty. On the first chart, place a dot opposite the appropriate score at each time interval. On the second chart, tick the appropriate pulse and breathing rates at each interval.

LEVEL OF RESPONSE CHART

DATE.............................. CASUALTY'S NAME..................................

OBSERVATION	RESPONSE/SCORE	Time of observation (minutes)					
		0	10	20	30	40	50
Eyes Observe for reaction while testing other responses.	Open spontaneously 4 Open to speech 3 Open to painful stimulus 2 No response 1						
Speech When testing responses, speak clearly and directly, close to casualty's ear.	Responds sensibly to questions 5 Seems confused 4 Uses inappropriate words 3 Incomprehensible sounds 2 No response 1						
Movement Apply painful stimulus: pinch ear lobe or skin on back of hand.	Obeys commands 6 Points to pain 5 Withdraws from stimulus 4 Bends limbs in response to pain 3 Straightens limbs in response to pain 2 No response 1						
	TOTAL SCORE						

PULSE AND BREATHING CHECK CHART

DATE.............................. CASUALTY'S NAME..................................

PULSE/BREATHING	RATE	Time of observation (minutes)					
		0	10	20	30	40	50
Pulse (beats per minute) Take pulse at wrist or at neck on adult, or at inner arm on baby (p.8). Note the rate, and whether beats are weak (w) or strong (s), regular (reg) or irregular (irreg).	Over 110						
	101–110						
	91–100						
	81–90						
	71–80						
	61–70						
	Below 61						
Breathing (breaths per minute) Note rate, and whether breathing is quiet (q) or noisy (n), easy (e) or difficult (diff).	Over 40						
	31–40						
	21–30						
	11–20						
	Below 20						
	TOTAL SCORE						